The
Five-Elements Wellness Plan

*A Chinese System
for Perfect Health*

BARBARA TEMELIE

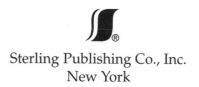

Sterling Publishing Co., Inc.
New York

LIBRARY OF CONGRESS CATALOGING-IN-PUBLICATION DATA

10 9 8 7 6 5 4 3 2 1

Published by Sterling Publishing Company, Inc.
387 Park Avenue South, New York, N.Y. 10016
© 2002 by Barbara Temelie
Distributed in Canada by Sterling Publishing
c/o Canadian Manda Group, One Atlantic Avenue, Suite 105
Toronto, Ontario, Canada M6K 3E7
Distributed in Great Britain and Europe by Cassell PLC
Wellington House, 125 Strand, London WC2R 0BB, England
Distributed in Australia by Capricorn Link (Australia) Pty. Ltd.
P.O. Box 704, Windsor, NSW 2756 Australia

TRANSLATION EDITED BY LAUREL ORNITZ

Sterling ISBN 0-8069-5867-7

Contents

Acknowledgments

With all my heart, I thank all my teachers, but especially Ole Nydahl. I also want to acknowledge and thank the Chinese doctor and qigong therapist Dr. Zheng Bin Zhang; my friend Martin Bruckmeier, a medical doctor in TCM, specializing in healing with qigong, in Chengdu, China, who made it possible for me to experience everyday Chinese cooking and its wonderful effects; my training-group colleagues, my friends Gabriele Klinger, Susanne Peroutka, and Christiane Seifert, for being there for me and for our productive, joyful, and engaged teamwork; my German editor Erdmute Otto, for the inspiring, helpful exchange of ideas; and the illustrator Tomek Twardowski, for the creative, harmonious communication during the conversion of ideas into images; and, at Sterling in New York, acquisitions editor Sheila Barry, for finding this book and having faith in it, and my editor Laurel Ornitz, whose editorial skill was enhanced by her knowledge of holistic medicine, her stylistic sense, and her empathy and enthusiasm for the subject.

Preface

When I wrote this book in 1992, few Westerners were aware of the centuries-old traditional Chinese diet, upon which the Five-Elements Wellness Plan is based. Therefore, I decided to write a book about the principles of Chinese dietetics, which are not only timeless but also applicable everywhere. I wrote this book for people who are concerned about their own nutrition in addition to therapists in the field of traditional Chinese medicine. As the book spread over the German-speaking countries of Europe, many people became interested in learning about Chinese medicine to the extent to be able to diagnose imbalances and recommend food according to the Five-Elements Plan. Now, with this version of the book in English, I am happy to pass the treasures of this nutritional system on to you.

In studying traditional Chinese medicine twenty years ago, I became acquainted with Chinese dietetics as a preventive or healing therapy practiced by doctors in China. I then learned that Chinese people all over the world select their food and cook their meals according to its principles. For instance, they use certain vegetables, grains, or spices to cool down the body in cases of heat, say, to overcome sleeping problems. Or they use a particular dish including lamb and hot spices to strengthen their defense mechanism. To be able to enhance vitality, prevent disease, or support a therapy in cases of illness simply by eating a certain way seemed very compelling to me, causing me to investigate this further.

I came to believe that a basic understanding of Chinese physiology and pathology would be necessary in order for people to be able to evaluate their particular constitution and, based upon that, to determine which foods are beneficial or therapeutic for them. One of my goals, therefore, was to simplify the Chinese understanding of health and disease so that it would be intelligible to Westerners. I was also concerned with the question regarding how the principles of Chinese dietetics could be put into practice in the West.

According to Chinese dietetics, the traditional way of eating, as it has been practiced over generations, should be modified only as much as necessary to adapt it to present needs. This is because, for thousands of years, human beings have created all kinds of enzymes and established the physiological systems of digestion and metabolism based upon the foods that they have eaten.

At the same time, I was wondering if the Chinese principles are universal—that is, whether or not the same principles regarding healthy food could be found in other cultures. In the West, are there traditions that took into account the energetic effect of food as well as its healing properties, and can this be seen today in the regional dishes you find all over the world?

My natural instinct for good food guided me to the right restaurants and to the right people throughout Europe, America, and Asia, where I was traveling as a nutritional consultant giving seminars. Thus, I was able to amass a great deal of information about the art of cooking simple dishes in bustling, fast-paced cultures. What I discovered after many years was that the traditional dishes of all the cultures I visited did in fact reflect knowledge regarding the energetic effect of food. I also saw that these dishes were passed on one generation to the next in order to satisfy the inherited physiological needs of the people.

However, I found Western classical principles of healthy cooking to be documented very poorly. Thus, I held to the principles of Chinese dietetics and devised a nutritional system based on it, as well as on diagnosis according to traditional Chinese medicine and on Chinese medicine in general.

This system, which became known as the "Five-Elements Plan," is modernized in some ways but essentially the same as its predecessor in its fundamental principles. The Five-Elements Plan truly offers satisfaction, not only when it comes to the superficial hunger of the stomach but also the hunger of each organ and each cell.

According to traditional Chinese medicine, among the organs the heart receives the best part of each meal. Selected by the stomach, the aroma of the food goes to the heart to nourish it. We are bound to have a good appetite and to enjoy our meal as well as the good company around the table, when the aromas come from a meal that is fresh and tasty and made with natural ingredients and spices. Thus, the art of cooking is a very old and natural way of bringing joy and good relationships into our lives, both of which are highly esteemed in China and viewed as basic conditions for health and longevity.

—BARBARA TEMELIE

Introduction

First, let me dispel some common myths: As oranges are high in vitamin C, many people eat them especially in the winter to prevent or fight off head colds or the flu. But did you know that oranges actually weaken the immune system? Bananas, on the other hand, are particularly high in potassium. However, were you aware that eating bananas often leads to fatigue and poor concentration, and can obstruct the lungs with phlegm, especially in small children? Yogurt and cottage cheese are common staples in many weight-loss diets, but did you know that they are not really helpful in losing weight? And what could be more invigorating than drinking ice-cold water on a hot summer day? Yet this actually leads to an overall weakening of vitality, as life energy is decreased, weight is gained as a result of poor digestion, and there is a lowering of libido.

In China, people were shocked when I told them that in the West we drink ice-cold beverages out of the refrigerator and allow children to have ice cream and other cooling foods like tomatoes even in the winter. Then I explained that Westerners are not familiar with the concept of the *thermal effects of foods,* a basic component of the Five-Elements Plan. When the thermal nature of foods is taken into account in our daily nutrition, benefits can be seen in just a few days. In the long run, selecting and preparing foods according to their thermal effect will support our efforts to remain slim and become healthier and more vital.

In the pages that follow, not only will you find out about the properties and the qualities of good, healthy food, but you will also learn how to sense the needs of your own body and get a feeling for what is good for you. Far from being another fad diet, the Five-Elements Plan is based upon the ancient principles of traditional Chinese medicine (TCM). Unchanged, these principles are still being followed today in China, in kitchens, restaurants, and hospitals. What is presented here is an adapted and modernized version of the traditional Chinese diet, with pivotal consequences for:

- @ All those who have tried to eat healthily and consciously but have again and again reached the limits of conventional diets.
- @ Those who have taken individual substances like minerals, vitamins, and enzymes to give them more vitality and strength and improve their health, but with little visible results.
- @ People who want to take responsibility for their own health.
- @ Those who would like to trust the reactions of their own bodies to guide them to a diet that is right for them.
- @ People who enjoy life and want to know how they can balance a rich meal at home or at a restaurant the next day.
- @ Very busy people—they can cook according to the Five-Elements Plan without spending a lot of time, or they can select a meal at a restaurant according to this system.
- @ People who are suspicious of the food produced by the conventional food industry.

@ People who are looking for a holistic nutrition system, where eating habits are changed step-by-step.

If you were to ask me which food is the most beneficial for all conditions, I would not be able to answer your question, as each food has a certain property and activates a certain process in the body. But answering the same question regarding beverages is easy. It is China's oldest beverage since the use of fire, and it was sold there everywhere on the streets long before the Chinese discovered green tea, which is their national beverage today. This mysterious drink has exceptional therapeutic benefits and can be used for any kind of indisposition, from lovesickness to stomachaches to headaches to menstrual cramps, making medication often unnecessary. It is also a good antidote to coldness and indigestion, and even helps if you are overweight.

It can be prepared easily, and you can take it with you everywhere in a thermos. There are absolutely no unpleasant side effects, and it can basically be substituted for all other beverages. The recommended dosage is from half a quart (or liter) to 2 quarts (or liters) a day. A cup before going to bed is especially good for your health and relaxing. And, by the way, it's almost free. If you haven't guessed what beverage I'm referring to, I will gladly tell you: *hot water!* Here's another tip: Should you want to order hot water at a restaurant, and after repeating yourself several times, the waiter still doesn't get it, try saying, "I would like to have a cup of tea without the teabag."

Chinese Dietetics in the West

The increasing dissatisfaction with Western medicine has produced some positive phenomena. Many people are now taking responsibility for their own health; the result is more conscious eating and a growing need for information about food.

The development of an increasingly high-tech health system has not stopped the decline in the overall population's state of health. Many people disappointed by conventional Western medicine can be seen in the offices of nonmedical practitioners and at health seminars. This in turn has had an effect on the established health system. Those people who make decisions are now being forced to reconsider various alternative approaches, as many doctors' practices are empty, results of therapy are poor, and medical costs are exploding. Such reevaluation brings about changes in society. Formerly, you'd be smiled at and regarded as an "air head" if you trusted in the Eastern healing arts and frequented health-food stores. Today, professors of medicine teach traditional Chinese medicine at universities, and many renowned institutions strongly advocate a more healthy way of living. In addition, a large number of individual patients are pressuring health-insurance companies to pay for alternative healing methods, which will ultimately save costs. Unfortunately, many insurance companies have yet to comply with their wishes.

Nevertheless, dissatisfaction with the existing system leads steadily to more openness to new development.

Today, you can chose from a wide range of natural healing methods, including Chinese dietetics. This ancient nutritional system has been tested extensively, and numerous empirical studies at large university hospitals in China have proven its efficacy. Furthermore, it distinguishes itself through being able to be applied so easily. Even when selecting a meal at a restaurant, you can follow its guidelines. This system is extremely compatible, meaning that its principles can be applied in any culture and in any climate. You need neither especially exotic ingredients nor excellent cooking skills. And you'll be able to forgo calculating calories, nutritive values, minerals, vitamins, and so forth, which can kill the appetite. If you are one of those people who are completely confused by the barrage of diets for health or losing weight, and if you don't know anymore what to eat because of so much often conflicting information, you will find a real alternative in Chinese dietetics.

Most diets and systems of nutrition are based on the assumption that the individual ingredients of a food have a positive influence on certain body functions. It is undisputed that this assumption is correct. But the sum of the individual effects does not tell us anything about the overall effect.

What is the effect of the food as a whole, as a living unity, on the human organism? Do you feel well after a meal, or are you tired and unable to concentrate? Is your digestion functioning well enough, or are you troubled by that feeling of being too full and by flatulence? Is your body temperature comfortable, or are you cold? Does the way you eat protect you from head colds and allergies, or do you have a weak immune system? And, finally, do you feel good about your body, or are you, for example, unhappy about being overweight? The problems mentioned here can be eradicated by adhering to the principles of a healthy and holistic nutritional system, as their causes can be found mainly in the imbalance of today's eating habits. Individual substances cannot solve these problems. If that were the case, the common cold would have died out in the West a long time ago, considering the enormous amount of vitamin C absorbed when eating oranges and other types of tropical fruit.

In fact, not only are individual substances ineffective in eliminating certain symptoms, but they can also lead to additional health problems. Because certain vitamins and minerals are praised so highly, many people are enticed to consume large amounts of particular groups of food or individual foods high in these vitamins and minerals. For example, when eaten regularly, tropical fruit, such as bananas, and milk products, especially for small children, cause digestive problems, loss of energy, and decreased performance ability, as well as weakening of the immune system. Later in this book, their connections will be explained. But for now remember to avoid eating an unbalanced diet, which causes deficiencies, by consuming a wide range of foods and by selecting fresh food that is in season. People today who eat "normally" are often healthier than many a disciple of the various fad diets, as these new approaches are frequently unbalanced and neglect the energetic effect of food on the individual.

In the West, there is also a long history of proponents of natural cures who took into account the holistic and energetic effects of nutrition. For example, Hildegard von Bingen, a Catholic nun who lived in Germany in the twelfth century, was an expert on the healing value of herbs, and many miraculous cures are attributed to her.

And the ancient Greek physician, Hippocrates, known as the father of medicine, emphasized the influence of diet and the patient's general way of living on his health and convalescence. But by and large, such supporters of a holistic approach were limited in their opportunities to further develop their knowledge along these lines.

Analysis of scientific research took over the responsibility for the health of the human being. And while the focus of scientists became smaller and smaller, the energy in nutrition and the overall health of people seemed to fall by the wayside.

Traditional Chinese Medicine

For three thousand years, traditional Chinese medicine has made use of a holistic nutritional system to preserve health and to heal existing disturbances. Over the course of the past three millennia, it's been proven that this nutritional system actually maintains health and balances unstable functions of the body. In addition, along with the other therapeutic methods of TCM—acupuncture, herbal therapy, and physiotherapy—traditional Chinese dietetics has been found to play an important role in the prevention of illness. Nevertheless, Chinese dietetics is still unknown for the most part in the West.

The first Westerners confronted with the art of healing in China were missionaries, followed by adventure-seeking scientists. Certainly, the most spectacular phenomenon of Chinese medicine that these early travelers to the East saw was acupuncture. This is the practice of puncturing the body with needles at specific points to cure disorders or relieve pain. Anyone who has seen a film of an operation in a Chinese hospital can attest to its lasting impression. While the doctors are performing open surgery, the patient, who is anaesthetized through acupuncture, can be seen talking to the nurse! It is not surprising that acupuncture was foremost in stirring the curiosity of Western researchers and that books specializing in this treatment were translated first. Nobody particularly noticed that a patient with a certain disorder was prescribed a special herb or that a young mother, right after giving birth, was prescribed chicken soup, which had been simmering for several days.

Besides being less dramatic, Chinese dietetics may have caught on in the West less than acupuncture for another important reason. Until a few years ago, the church and science were basically the domains of men. It's likely that neither the missionaries nor the scientists thought it worthwhile to even mention the wonderful effects of hearty soups and herbal teas. So, how could Westerners have learned about them? Yet, one particular Chinese healing herb that has since become famous throughout the West did catch the male travelers' attention: the ginseng root. Could its potency-enhancing effect have triggered their interest?

In China, herbal therapy and nutrition are closely intertwined. In daily life in hospitals as well as in private kitchens, healing herbs are often cooked in meals. For example, you will frequently find the slightly bitter-tasting dong-quai root in chicken soup. Chicken soup nourishes the body and stimulates the production of bodily fluids. The dong-quai root builds up blood. When both are combined, a simple soup turns into a delicious, blood-strengthening remedy. Thus, for the Chinese people, food is not only enjoyed for its taste, but is also regarded as a means of specifically strengthening health. The art of cooking therefore takes on a very high standard in China.

It is important to distinguish between therapeutic nutrition and daily nutrition. The goal of this book is to make the general guiding principles of both accessible. Therapeutic principles can be applied only when a diagnosis based on traditional Chinese medicine has been made. Since the beginning of Chinese dietetics, many tourists have walked over the Chinese wall, yet the eating habits of the Chinese have basically remained the same. The principles of nutrition followed in ancient times are still being applied daily today and with the same success. Therefore, it can rightfully be said that Chinese dietetics has evolved from the most successful and tested nutritional system we know. Much would be gained if food prepared not only in private kitchens and restaurants but especially in hospitals were inspired by this form of nutrition.

Is he a cook or a doctor?
Is this a pharmacy or a restaurant?
Fish, meat, vegetables, spring onion, and leek:
Delicious meals prohibit tablets and pills,
Nourishing dishes are the remedy for all kinds of suffering

—CHINESE POEM OF UNKNOWN ORIGIN

The Chinese Philosophy
of Long Life

It can be said that the striving for technical progress has characterized the development of Western civilization. In China, it was the striving for immortality, or at least very long life, that produced an array of cultural achievements, including TCM and with it Chinese dietetics. China owes this development to Taoism, a mystical philosophy that drew its knowledge from the observation of nature and from the understanding of cosmic connections. It is often said that its most famous teacher Lao-tzu, who lived in the sixth century B.C., was its founder. But actually the roots of Taoism go back to a period thousands of years before that, and are lost in time.

According to Taoism's Doctrine of Changes, there is no static state in the universe; everything is moving constantly. If a state seems to be static, it is merely because the process of formation or of disintegration is so slow that we cannot perceive it. If we observe a stone or a mountain range over the course of a couple of years, they seem to be static; there is no visible change. But after a longer period of time, we can clearly see a difference. Changes like this in nature do not take place in a matter of years but rather over millions of years.

We human beings, as well, are constantly subjected to a process of change, and we are basically uncertain as to what the future will bring. In order to escape from this existential uncertainty, people have tried to recognize the laws according to which changes occur. If we understand what is happening, it becomes predictable, can be calculated, and loses its threat. Fear of the unknown in human existence is an important impetus in producing philosophies, religions, culture, and technical progress.

In China, the longing for salvation from the terrors of human existence—misfortunes, illnesses, and death— produced Taoism. The goals of the Taoist disciples were to develop wisdom and to gain an understanding of the origin of existence. They had to spend a great deal of time on mental exercises in order to reach enlightenment. As Taoists attribute less importance to rebirth than Buddhists do (Buddhism came to China only in the fourth century B.C.), their highest objective over time became achieving immortality or very old age. (For the Chinese, "immortality" is synonymous with the Buddhist term "enlightenment.") Living to an old age would give them the time needed to practice meditation and other mental exercises in order to achieve a high level of spiritual development, which is always accompanied by the highest joy.

Soon striving for a long life had developed its own dynamics and reaching old age in health had become an end in itself and a fixed idea in the minds of the Chinese people. The numerous meditative exercises for health purposes, as well as exercises in physical therapy, that developed in China are proof of this fixation on longevity. Among them, *tai chi ch'uan,* recognized for its slow, flowing, circular movements, is perhaps the best known. The other methods of TCM—acupuncture, herbal and nutritional therapy, and especially diagnosis—were critically influenced by this new goal. The aim of a long life challenged the diagnostic abilities of doctors and added pressure to not allowing pathological processes to develop in the first place. This went hand in hand with the development of a comprehensive understanding of the causes of illness.

A wealth of medical knowledge and experience was preserved within families of doctors as secret knowledge and was handed down from one generation to the next. This tradition, a consequence of the political and social structure of China, made sure that medical theories and principles were kept pure and correct, but it did little in the way of providing medical benefits for the common people.

Prevention, the most important tenet of TCM, requires special skills when it comes to recognizing pathological processes early on. Medical diagnosis makes it possible to recognize illnesses, or, to put it more precisely, an imbalance, before serious symptoms have developed. By feeling the pulse at the wrist at six different spots on two levels, precise evaluations can be made about the condition of the twelve organs and about the overall constitution of the person. Another very important diagnostic method is through carefully examining the tongue: its color, form, moisture, and mobility, as well as the color and condition of its coating. By asking the patient questions and by closely observing the patient's face and body, the overall picture is completed. This is the practical way of proceeding before giving therapeutic nutritional advice for prevention or treatment of an illness.

However, something else is required for detecting pathological changes early on that involves another way of looking at things. The stomach is not only ill when it hurts. The illness process has already been going on for some time before stomach pains develop. Before a heart attack happens, the ill person has probably been suffering for quite a while from ailments like troubled sleep or inner restlessness, which may indicate an illness of the heart. Many people complain about such things as troubled sleep, inner restlessness, nausea, constipation, being over-weight, tiredness, lack of concentration, and other "functional disturbances." There are pills for all of these problems, and hardly anybody inquires about their causes. The connection between a symptom, which seems commonplace at first, and an illness, which may turn serious later, is often not recognized. Traditional Chinese diagnosis does not work wonders in this respect; it merely asks about origins and recognizes connections. To further understand these connections, it is necessary to look at the Chinese way of viewing the human body.

What Is Illness?

Life is essentially based on two components: energy and matter. If one of the two components exists excessively or insufficiently, the person is ill. If one component is missing altogether, there is no life. Death means that energy and matter are separating from each other. With this understanding, we have already entered into the Chinese way of thinking, based on the *yin-yang* model.

According to TCM, yin and yang represent opposing yet complementary aspects of the universe. Everything can be thought of in terms of a preponderance of either yin or yang. Vital energy, called "qi" by the Chinese (pronounced "chee"), has a *yang* character, as does everything that is bright, light, and directed upward and to the outside. The daytime and the sun, as well as anything that is masculine, active, nonmaterial, invisible, or incomprehensible, can be said to be yang. Matter has a *yin* character, as does everything dark, shady, and directed downward and to the inside. Examples are the night and the moon, as well as anything feminine, preserving, material, visible, or comprehensible.

Qi and matter are like fire and water. They control each other. Fire can evaporate water, and water can extinguish fire. The harmonious interplay of both poles ensures in a healthy organism a balanced temperature and dynamics. Imbalance means, in this sense, too hot or too cold, too dry or too damp, or too fast or too slow.

In the terminology of Chinese medicine, the yang factor (energy) is always called "qi." The terms "fluids" and

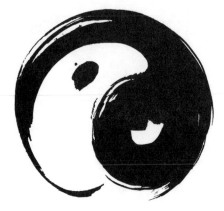

*The yin-yang model: Yang is qi, the light, the day, the sun, the male, the active,
the immaterial, the invisible, the incomprehensible. Yin is matter, the dark, the
night, the moon, the female, the preserving, the material, the visible, the
comprehensible.*

"blood" are commonly used for the yin factor (matter),
when it comes to expressing the polarity of yin and yang on
the level of the body. Sometimes references are made to qi
and blood and other times to qi and fluids.

The Yang of the Body

On the physical level, yang means qi and warmth, as well as
everything that keeps the organism alive with all its functions; all feelings, thoughts, and everything spiritual are
included in it as well. Basically, everything that is invisible
that has to do with the state of being alive is yang.

The first stage of a shortage in the realm of yang is
called a "deficiency of qi." Among other things, a deficiency
of qi expresses itself through fatigue and poor concentration. A deficiency of qi and warmth is worse than merely a
deficiency of qi, and is called a "deficiency of yang." It has
all the symptoms of the deficiency of qi but, in addition,
expresses itself with cold sensations like shivering and cold
feet, as well as mental and physical exhaustion. Too much

yang, or an "excess of yang," makes itself known through a sensation of heat, reddish skin color, an outburst of rage, or excessive activity.

In the event of an imbalance, we either deal with an excess or a deficiency of yang or with a deficiency of qi (there is no qi excess, except for qi that is blocked). In the language of Chinese medicine, the first case would be expressed this way: "The yang is in excess." A deficiency of yang or qi would be phrased, "The yang or the qi are weakened." Or one could say generally, "The *yang root* of the person is disturbed."

The Yin of the Body

The terms "blood," "fluids," and "matter" are used to describe the yin of the body. Everything that is substantial is included here: bodily fluids, blood, bones, tissue, muscles, brain mass, and so forth; in other words, everything that is visible. When the yin root of the person is disturbed, there is a deficiency of blood, a deficiency of yin, or an excess of yin.

An excess of yin is an accumulation of moisture in the body, which is called "dampness" in Chinese medicine and not to be equated with the good bodily fluids. In this case, water is retained in the tissue, which leads to swollen and heavy limbs, and the bronchial tubes fill up with mucus. Furthermore, with an excess of yin, one can become overweight, develop cellulite, and suffer from fatigue and depression.

The first stage of a deficiency of the yin root is a deficiency of blood. This diagnosis has a different meaning in Chinese medicine from that in conventional Western medicine. It refers not only to a reduction in the amount of blood but also in the functioning and in the quality of the blood. A deficiency of blood is less profound than a deficiency of yin, and essentially results in the eyes becoming sensitive to light, the face turning pale, and a tendency to develop muscle cramps.

A deficiency of yin, on the other hand, will result in dryness, as the bodily fluids are depleted. One then becomes restless and nervous as well as sometimes thin and emaciated. Skin and hair tend to be dry. There is frequently a problem with sweating at night, troubled sleep, and hot feet. With women, the unpleasant signs of menopause—hot flashes, night sweats, and troubled sleep—point to a natural deficiency of yin, which causes menstruation to stop, so that women who are getting older will not keep on losing blood or getting pregnant.

The examples mentioned here offer a general, rough view of the way Chinese medicine comprehends illness. In practice, it is the task of diagnosis to determine any imbalance between yin and yang in *every individual organ.* An imbalance in an organ has occurred when there is too much or too little yin or yang, or when qi stagnates. Because all the internal organs are connected with one another and depend on one another, health means a harmonious collaboration of the organs based on a balanced supply of qi and fluids.

As we are constantly subjected to internal and external ups and downs, balancing is a perpetual process in a healthy organism. When an organ is in a state of excess or deficiency for a short period of time, the other organs restore the balance by supplying or removing qi and fluids. A healthy diet, which ensures a balanced supply of qi and fluids, has the effect of keeping the internal fluctuations within permissible levels. On this basis, the body's mechanism for regulation is capable of balancing a short-term strain that produces a deficiency or excess in any organ.

How Does the Body Protect Itself from Illness?

An illness is always an excess or a deficiency of yang (qi and warmth) or yin (fluids and blood) in one or several organs. Just as the blood flows in the blood vessels, the qi flows through specific channels called "meridians." But qi also circulates freely in the body. The flow of qi and the flow of blood are closely connected, supporting or obstructing each other, depending on whether the body is open or blocked. The meridians and the blood vessels connect the various internal organs. Qi and blood flow through them, as in an electrical circuit, from organ to organ.

Blood nourishes, cools, and moistens the body. Blood gives us mental calmness, composure, and the ability to relax and sleep well. Regeneration and restful sleep rely on good blood. Qi energizes, transports, excretes, and warms. But its most important function is to convert substances that are foreign to the body, like food, so that they can be assimilated. This "metabolism" function and the excretion of waste material, which occur in every transformation process, such as digestion, can work only with the help of qi.

Qi activates us and produces impulses. It is also the substance out of which the heart creates joy. Depending upon its task, it receives different names. If it takes care of resistance, it is called "wei qi" (resistance energy). Wei qi protects the organism from contagious diseases and from climatic influences. It doesn't flow in the meridians, but circulates freely in and around the body.

In traditional Chinese medicine, there are five pairs of organs: liver and gallbladder, heart and small intestine, spleen and stomach, lungs and large intestine, kidneys and bladder. In this sequence, called the "generative cycle," the organs are supplied with qi by means of circulation through the meridians.

A pair always consists of one yin and one yang organ. The first in the pair is the yin organ, followed by the yang organ. The yin organs, also called "storage organs," provide qi and yin. The yang organs, also known as "hollow organs," are involved with intake, excretion, digestion, and transport.

In cases of any impediment, in which more blood or qi is used, the organ is protected doubly. The partner organ always strives to balance the deficiency of its partner, by giving it some of its qi or blood, and the organ pair situated in front of it does the same. If, for example, there is a deficiency of qi in the spleen, the stomach will support the spleen, and the heart-and-small-intestine pair will supply more qi to the spleen as well, in order to reestablish the balance. Thus, short-term disturbances are balanced in a healthy organism, even before ailments occur.

The above description is an oversimplification of the complex cooperation that takes place among the organs. However, because of these close connections, disorders— as well as positive influences—will affect several organs or the entire organism in a short period of time. Therefore, a balanced diet is the best protection from illness, as the qi and blood buildup that takes place from eating high-quality food ensures that the organs will be well supplied and can execute the balancing process in cases of any disturbance to the organism.

How Does Illness Come About?

In the chapter about the five elements, the causes of illness are examined in detail. In general, however, traditional Chinese medicine distinguishes between *internal* and *external* factors that make us ill. Internal factors have to do with emotions and mental concepts; external ones include climatic influences, other environmental forces, and diet. The imbalance that can be caused by these factors manifests as states of *excess* or *deficiency*, but also as a blockage in the flow of qi, called "qi stagnation."

Disorders that primarily concern qi and yang are called "illnesses of the yang root." Within the yang root, the following pathological processes occur: a deficiency of qi, a deficiency of yang, and an excess of yang. In this context, yang stands for warmth or heat. A deficiency of qi is the first stage in the development of illness, and it is indicative of a loss of energy. A deficiency of yang indicates a loss of qi and warmth or a state of coldness. An excess of yang implies that there is too much heat in the body, and this eventually causes the bodily fluids to dry up; it can also lead to a deficiency of yin.

Disorders that mainly concern yin are called "illnesses of the yin root." Within the yin root, the following pathological developments take place: a deficiency of blood, a deficiency of yin, and an excess of yin. These conditions develop over the course of years, so there are gradual gradations in the seriousness of the condition. In comparison to a deficiency of yin, a deficiency of blood is often less serious. A deficiency of yin begins with a lack of bodily fluids and can develop to a point where it causes real damage. Then, emaciation, hair loss, osteoporosis (decalcification of the bones), brittleness of the bones, and cardiovascular diseases can occur.

An excess of yin indicates excessive dampness in the body, which becomes evident as water retention in the tissue. Being overweight always points to an excess of yin. The condition of dampness signifies that digestion and metabolism are working inadequately and that waste material is not being excreted sufficiently, so waste and toxins build up in the body, accumulating in the tissues. In addition, dampness can develop into thick phlegm, leading to hot conditions as well as severe chronic illnesses.

Balance

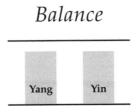

Yang root and yin root in balance = health

A balance between the yin and yang roots equals health. When blood, fluids, and matter are sufficient, our nerves are calm and we are able to regenerate through relaxation and restful sleep. Sufficient qi and warmth take care of our vitality and protection. In addition, there are no problems with lack of libido or sexual potency.

Yang-Root Weakness

In a healthy organism, yin and yang support and control each other. On one side of the scale are qi and warmth. As long as there is enough qi and warmth, an excessive increase in yin is not possible. However, if qi and warmth are reduced in the body, due to cold weather, overexertion, or cooling foods, a weakness of the yang root occurs. This results in a deficiency of qi or a deficiency of yang and is often accompanied by an excess of yin (dampness). Whether we manifest a qi or a yang deficiency, with or without an excess of yin, depends on trigger factors and on our constitution. Signs of a deficiency of qi, a deficiency of yang, and an excess of yin follow.

Qi Deficiency

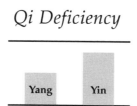

A deficiency of qi: The yang root is lowered, and the yin root is normal.

- General weakness
- Fatigue after a meal
- Poor concentration
- Craving for sweet food
- Feeling of being too full, flatulence
- Possibly lack of appetite
- Loose, shapeless stools
- Food sensitivities
- Weak immunity
- Cold hands

Yang Deficiency

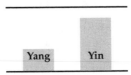

A deficiency of yang: The yang root is lowered a great deal, and the yin root is normal.

- @ Exhaustion
- @ Mental fatigue
- @ Lack of drive
- @ Possibly anxieties, resignation
- @ Craving for sweet food
- @ Craving for coffee or Coke
- @ No recuperation through sleep
- @ Frequently feeling cold; cold feet, knees, hips, buttocks
- @ Having loose stools more than once a day
- @ Loose or watery stools containing undigested food
- @ Frequent urination, urination at night
- @ Light-colored urine
- @ Feeling of being too full, flatulence
- @ Menstrual cramps, which improve through warmth
- @ Pain in the lower back in the morning, which improves through movement
- @ Aversion to cold food and beverages
- @ Weak libido, possibly impotence

Yin Excess

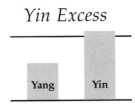

Yin excess (dampness): The yin root is increased excessively, and the yang root is lowered.

@ Heavy feeling in the arms and legs
@ Clumsiness
@ Mental and physical sluggishness
@ Dull feeling in the head
@ Being prone to head colds, with strong production of phlegm
@ Lack of thirst
@ Cold hands
@ Flatulence, feeling of being too full
@ Craving for coffee
@ Possibly visible water retention in the face, arms, or legs
@ Tendency to be depressed
@ Possibly being overweight

In each of these three conditions, all or only a few of the listed signs can occur, or they can be combined. Also, it is normal, even for healthy people, to occasionally exhibit any of the listed complaints and for them to disappear on their own.

Please be aware that these lists are not sufficient for making a proper diagnosis — neither for yourself nor for other people. They can merely point you in the direction of the beginning of an illness and perhaps help you recognize a tendency toward either heat, coldness, or dampness, so that you can choose the foods most suitable.

Case Study:
Qi Deficiency of the Spleen with Dampness (Yin Excess)

This case study involves a twenty-four-year-old woman who sits down all day at her job and has been overweight for years. Apart from some short-term successes, all diets she has been on have actually exacerbated her weight problem. She has also been suffering for some months from fatigue, especially after meals, and from the feeling of being overly full and from flatulence. Although she has a strong craving for both sweets and coffee, she is hardly ever thirsty. Her hands are often cold, and she gets cold easily. Over the past few months, she has had water retention in her face early in the morning after getting up, and she has spoken of feeling depressed.

She told me that in her childhood she had a dessert consisting mainly of cottage cheese every day after lunch. Her mother favored milk products in general. Her weight problems can be attributed to a deficiency of qi in the spleen, brought on by the dampening and cooling effect of the milk products (the thermal effects of foods will be discussed in greater detail later). Her body didn't have enough qi and warmth to burn the food, so fat and water accumulated in the tissue. The diets she went on later, in which tropical fruit, which also cool the body, played a major role, worsened the situation.

The spleen is the "ruler over the fluids." It distributes the bodily fluids and transports excess fluids to the excretory organs. As time went on, she developed a chronic deficiency of qi and dampness in the spleen, so these tasks were not being handled properly anymore. The result was water retention in her face and depression. Overall, the chronic deficiency of qi resulted in a reduction of warmth energy, a slowdown of metabolism, and an accumulation of dampness (yin excess).

Yin-Root Weakness

The three conditions and the case study above are examples of a weakness of the yang root. Now let's have a look at the reverse situation: a weakness of the yin root, meaning a decrease of yin and an increase of yang. Do you remember the disorders of the yin root? Deficiencies of blood and yin indicate dryness, and yang in excess points to heat. Here, it's important to mention the close connection between these two roots. A deficiency of blood usually goes hand in hand with a deficiency of qi in the spleen, as the spleen supplies the utilizable essence from the food, from which the organism produces blood. Or, put differently, a deficiency of blood is a result of a spleen qi deficiency in most cases. Understanding this connection is important for our selection of food. In cases where there is a deficiency of blood, nutritional recommendations, above all, include foods that strengthen the qi of the spleen. Thus, the spleen is able to produce blood out of refreshing, moistening food, which is also recommended to build up blood.

A deficiency of yin (a lack of bodily fluids) involves a process of drying out. In this case, as far as nutrition is concerned, it's a matter of not only strengthening yin but the spleen's qi as well, so that bodily fluids can be produced. Whereas a deficiency of blood concerns the liver and the heart, a deficiency of yin involves the liver, the heart, the stomach, the lungs, the large intestine, and/or the kidneys.

We've already covered the excess of yin in connection with the disorders of the yang root, as an excess of yin is based on a weakness of the yang root. Now we will deal with the excess of yang. This condition, often connected with yin weakness, can be balanced by means of dietary therapy through strengthening of the yin root. Whether, over the course of a drying-out or heating process, a blood weakness, a yin deficiency, or an excess of yang comes about depends on the triggering factors and on the constitution of the person concerned.

Blood Deficiency

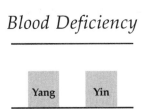

A blood deficiency: The yin root and the yang root are lowered, as a lack of blood usually results from a deficiency of qi.

- @ Sensitivity to light, swimming of the eyes, night blindness
- @ Limbs falling asleep
- @ Tendency toward muscle cramps
- @ Pale face
- @ Emotional vulnerability and being thin-skinned
- @ Emotional imbalance
- @ Fatigue due to mental or intellectual overexertion
- @ Difficulties falling asleep

Yin Deficiency

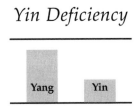

A deficiency of yin: The yin root is lowered a great deal, and the yang root is lowered, as a lack of yin is usually the result of a deficiency of qi. Nevertheless, due to dryness, signs of heat develop.

- @ Night sweats
- @ Hot feet, especially at night
- @ Thirst, a dry mouth
- @ Troubled sleep
- @ Internal feeling of heat
- @ Restlessness, nervousness
- @ Being prone to stress
- @ Little perseverance, little tolerance to stress
- @ Possibly dizziness
- @ Possibly thinness and emaciation

Yang Excess

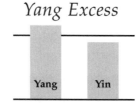

Excess of yang: The yang root is increased, and the yin root is lowered, as heat depletes yin.

- @ Hot sensations in the body
- @ Reddish face color
- @ Hyperactivity
- @ Dominating personality, loud voice
- @ Troubled sleep
- @ Strong thirst
- @ Desire for cold beverages and food
- @ Tendency to be irritated or angry
- @ Incompatibility with massage or psychological pressure
- @ Possibly voracious hunger

Case Study: Deficiency of Yin

This case study concerns a thirty-year-old architect who had been overtaxing himself for more than a year as he was developing his own business. For several months, he had been breaking out in sweat during the night, after finally having fallen asleep. In addition, in bed he needed to uncover his feet, because they felt so hot. He complained about being nervous, saying that stress was getting to him more than it used to. The first year of his self-employment was very exhausting. He often worked late into the night, drinking cup after cup of strong coffee the next day to stay awake.

It was apparent that he had a deficiency of fluids (yin deficiency) due to mental overexertion, stimulants like coffee, which are drying, and lack of sleep. A deficiency of yin is often seen in older people. But nowadays even many young people who work hard in their careers already show signs of suffering from it. These symptoms, however, usually disappear with improvements in their lifestyle and diet.

Satisfied with the results of his hard work over the past year, the architect felt that he could finally switch to a lower gear. After some weeks of sufficient sleep and an appropriate diet, his symptoms in fact disappeared.

When a short-term severe stress produces an imbalance, it is relatively easy to harmonize the condition, but only through the elimination of the triggering factors. The longer the stress lasts, the more profound the disorder and the more organs affected, and the longer it will take to reestablish the balance.

Important Note

The nutritional recommendations contained in the Five-Elements Plan above all can be applied in the prevention of illness. Furthermore, they can be used to balance an uncomplicated disorder, especially when the causes of the disorder are connected to improper diet. Doctors, nonmedical practitioners, and nutritionists who practice TCM use Chinese dietary therapy to strengthen health, relieve ailments, and cure illnesses.

The explanations in this book will make it possible for you to understand the formation of pathological processes and apply the principles of Chinese dietetics as a preventive measure. *But the information provided here is in no way sufficient for you to be able to make a diagnosis, in the sense of TCM, and to cure an illness.*

What Is the Role of a Diet Rich in Qi?

Let us first start by addressing these fundamental questions: From which sources does the body draw its qi, and how is it dispersed throughout the body? The organism is fed by two central energies: *prenatal qi* and *postnatal qi*. An energetic system called the "Triple Burner" spreads both throughout the organism to all the organs and the tissues. In the upper, middle, and lower levels of the organism, transformation processes are going on constantly that convert the intake of foreign matter, like food, air, and impressions, into something that will later build the body. The Upper Burner is associated with the heart and the lungs, the Middle Burner with the spleen and the stomach. The Lower Burner is the place where our resources of prenatal and postnatal qi are stored, and it is connected with the kidneys.

We bring prenatal qi with us when we are born. It consists of two components. One, made up of our parents' genotype, contains our genetic predisposition and cultural characteristics, such as our looks and culturally specific character traits. The other component is what is known as "cosmic qi." Depending on one's religious view, it is either seen as being of divine origin or as containing the spiritual impressions from former lives, so therefore of karmic origin.

Prenatal qi, stored in the kidneys, in the Lower Burner, is the basis of life. Our health, vitality, and life span depend, on the one hand, on the quantity of our prenatal qi and, on the other, on the quantity and the quality of our postnatal qi, which has the function of nourishing the body and activating the prenatal qi.

Certain problems can occur in connection with prenatal qi. If postnatal qi is deficient and prenatal qi thus cannot be activated, we lose vitality and age prematurely. When prenatal qi is depleted—for example, through an overextended lifestyle in combination with a poor diet and lack of sleep, or through taking drugs—the body as well as the mind will suffer and one's life span may even be shortened. Postnatal qi is our daily source of vitality, and it comes mainly from the food we eat. To feed postnatal qi means to preserve prenatal qi, which in turn influences the quality of our life and affects how long we live. This connection between qi and quality of life and longevity is the essential argument for a healthy and balanced diet.

The amount of prenatal qi that is available is determined from birth and cannot be replenished. So, the trick is to preserve it. All Chinese exercises for health, from movement arts like tai chi and qigong to Taoist practices and

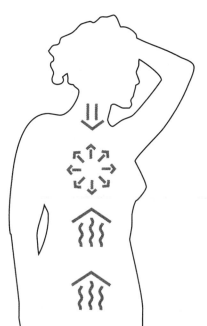

The production of postnatal qi out of food and the air we breathe

Breathing Qi is obtained through the lungs from the air that we breathe.
Upper Burner: *Rising nutrition qi mixes with breathing qi to become postnatal qi, which nourishes the organism.*
Middle Burner: *Nutrition qi is obtained with the help of the yang of the spleen from nutrition.*
Lower Burner: *The rising yang of the kidneys supports the transformation of nutrition in the Middle Burner.*

meditation exercises, and of course the art of healthy cooking, initially were intended to produce postnatal qi in order to keep the loss of prenatal qi as low as possible. Every day the kidneys relinquish, depending on the demand, a small amount of this prenatal qi to the organism, in order to sustain all the functions of the body. Consequently, we age due to the daily loss of prenatal qi.

Picture this: a basin, with a water bucket on one side and a glowing coal on the other, situated in the lower part of the body, below the navel *(Lower Burner, kidneys)*. Both water and fire, yin and yang, are contained in what is understood as prenatal qi. However, you'll note a slight discrepancy with the images here. According to what has been presented so far, the water bucket can be seen as yin, and qi has a yang character. Unfortunately, every now and then there are inconsistencies like this in TCM; this is just something we have to live with.

Prenatal qi is considered the basic "nutrition" for all organs and organ functions. In order to understand more precisely the functions of the Lower Burner that are important for life, the yin and yang of the kidneys need to be examined. Prenatal and postnatal qi feed the moist, nourishing, and cooling yin and the warming, activating yang of the kidneys. The yin of the kidneys is the foundation for the entire body's yin; similarly, the yang of the kidneys is the basis for the entire body's yang. The kidney yang is of critical importance for the function of digestion (see the illustration). Its rising fire warms and activates the Middle Burner and supports the yang of the spleen when food is digested.

The organs of the *Middle Burner,* the *spleen* and the *stomach,* are situated in the middle of the body. The rising kidney yang supplies them with strength and warmth, so that they can extract qi and fluids from food and make them available to the body. The function of the Middle Burner is to produce *nutrition qi* from what we eat. Of the two components that make up postnatal qi—nutrition qi and breathing qi—nutrition qi is the most important; this is how significant food is.

When the Lower and Middle Burners function well, the nutrition qi rises sufficiently into the upper part of the body so that it can feed the whole body and take care of the organs of the *Upper Burner,* the *lungs* and the *heart.* It is the task of the lungs to produce the second component of postnatal qi by extracting qi from the air that we breathe. This *breathing qi* mixes with the nutrition qi in the Upper Burner. The result is the creation of postnatal qi, an original form, which the body now transforms into all the qi forms: into blood, fluids, and substances the body needs.

The more postnatal qi is created, the less prenatal qi is used. However, if the organism is exposed to extreme stress—for example, due to polluted air, poor nutrition, drugs, illness, relationship problems, or an excessive lifestyle—little postnatal qi is produced. The output then exceeds the input; in other words, the expenses exceed the income, and the reserves—the prenatal qi—are eaten into. Thus, we can see from the role played by breathing qi and nutrition qi, that clean air and especially high-quality and nourishing food are crucial for the upkeep of the reserves.

The Subtle Flow of Qi

Essentially, it is the task of exercises for health like tai chi and qigong to improve breathing and the harmonious flow of qi. Thus, they have a balancing effect on the psyche, increasing our sense of well-being. Positive impressions in the mind, resulting from a compassionate attitude toward oneself and others, and emotional balance, in part the result of dealing mindfully with one's anger, play a large role in gaining qi and preserving it. The heart is the residence of the spirit, and the blood is its carrier. The heart is situated together with the lungs in the Upper Burner. Hot emotions like rage, anger, and aggression use up a lot of qi and end up depleting the bodily fluids. In addition, they disturb the subtle flow of qi. Exercises that improve breathing and harmonize the flow of qi have a calming and cooling effect on these fiery emotions.

On the other hand, cold emotions like fear, frustration, moodiness, avarice, and sadness block qi and the gaining of qi in the breathing organs, the digestive tract, and the area of the kidneys. Physical exercises that set qi in motion again and activate the organism are extremely helpful in this situation.

Lack of movement, perhaps due to a sedentary job, thus contributes to a deficiency of qi and to qi stagnation. The deficiency of qi among the organs essentially concerns the spleen and thus the powers of digestion, whereas qi stagnation is the result of a "tense" liver.

Liver qi stagnation makes itself known mostly in situations where there is conflict, often through a feeling of having a lump in one's throat. In women, it sometimes manifests before their periods in the form of premenstrual syndrome, with painful tension in the breasts as well as overall irritation and depression.

People who are under a great deal of time pressure and suffer from psychological tension as well, and for these and other reasons tend to eat a poor diet, often exhibit both a qi deficiency of the spleen and qi stagnation of the liver. Emotional stress, which tenses the liver, eventually obstructs digestion. This is the cause for an insufficient utilization of food, which in turn triggers such symptoms as feeling overly full and flatulence. In many cases, constipation, a tiresome subject and a more tiresome malady, can also be traced back to stagnation in the pathway of the liver.

Birth-control pills, taken by many women, are a further trigger for a spleen qi deficiency combined with liver qi stagnation, according to Bob Flaws, a gynecologist and TCM practitioner who has written several books on Chinese medicine and diet. In order to counterbalance such harmful side effects, relaxing physical exercise and a diet that especially strengthens the qi of the spleen are essential:

Every kind of movement and the activities we are engaged in during the day contribute to stimulating the production and the flow of qi. On the other hand, yin (blood and fluids) is produced during the night, basically while we sleep.

In order to activate the qi flow effectively and to loosen already existing blockages, it is recommended to take a three-pronged approach:

- By strengthening the qi of the spleen through a nourishing, wholesome, high-quality diet, you will protect the digestive tract from the blocking encroachments of the strained liver.
- By reducing the stress and the pressure in your life, the cause of the tension in the liver, you will be tackling the problem at its core.
- And third, through physical exercise without performance pressure, you will be able to decrease the tension in the pathway of the liver, which affects the entire organism and manifests mentally as a lack of flexibility. Aside from the Chinese methods of tai chi and qigong, physical movement and stretching exercises, sports without performance pressure, and walking, as well as taking the time to pursue creative interests, are ideal for loosening up physically, mentally, and emotionally.

In addition, a very simple way of releasing the qi of the liver and relaxing the liver is to lie down for five to ten minutes every now and then during the day.

Wholesome nourishment and a balance between activity and relaxation are crucial for health on the physical level. On the mental and emotional planes, it is important to have a positive outlook, to let go of negative moods and experiences, and to cultivate internal calmness. Without attending to the mental and emotional levels of our being, even if our diet is the best, puts us at risk of becoming ill, as the organism will not be capable of utilizing the offered nourishment and of excreting toxins. Therefore, it can be said that cultivating an open, cheery disposition, as well as being mindful regarding lifestyle decisions, play important roles in creating good health.

Ingredients and Digestibility

In cases of deficiency diseases, Western dietetics assumes that it is necessary to substitute the substances that the organism is lacking by supplying them from the outside. It is taken for granted that anything that is eaten ends up where it is needed. But this is not the case, and is an area that needs to be examined.

Digestibility, manifesting as the good feeling we get after a meal, is the critical sign that tells us that the nutrients have arrived where they are supposed to go. On the other hand, problems with digestion of any kind indicate that the food is being digested incompletely. Chinese dietetics, however, goes one critical step further. It is concerned with the food being of such a nature that its qi will be supplied to the internal organs, which require qi in order to function. In addition, the food that we eat has to strengthen the organs involved in digestion, so that the utilizable parts of the food can actually be absorbed.

One of the primary differences between Eastern and Western dietetics has to do with the issue of independence versus dependence. In Chinese dietetics, people are encouraged to perceive and judge for themselves what agrees with them and are shown ways to obtain what they need simply from their meals. Conversely, with the Western model, people are often dependent on food-value tables, calculations, and pills, and are basically not given any meaningful criteria by which to determine which foods they need.

What we eat, however, is not as important as how we digest it. In other words, it's better to eat a well-digested meal of poor quality than a poorly digested meal of high quality, when it comes to being sufficiently supplied with vital substances. Vegetables today contain less in the way of vital substances, or nutrients, than they did before industrialization, primarily because of overcultivation and pollution. Stress is another factor that increases the need for vital substances nowadays, to different degrees, according to the individual. It can be assumed that people who suffer from a tremendous amount of stress also don't eat a proper diet, another reason for a deficiency in nutrients. They often choose those foods that take the least time to prepare, such as frozen food, sandwiches, or meals they can heat up in the microwave oven, all of which lack sufficient qi and absorbable vital substances.

Supplementing food with vitamins and minerals may delay the harmful effects of exhaustion and a poor diet. Yet the benefits of supplements have yet to be proven scientifically, and some even have negative side effects, so they need to be taken with caution. If you eat a wide range of fresh foods, like all kinds of vegetables, potatoes, rice, small amounts of poultry, fish, and meat (or legumes in a vegetarian diet), with a variety of delicious and aromatic natural spices and herbs, it is very unlikely that you will require any supplements.

In the Five-Elements Plan, the emphasis is placed on foods in season, which have a strong aroma and are high in qi. Eating this way brings us a great variety over the year, and with variety we are assured of consuming an array of vital substances. Vital substances, not extracted, but as they are contained in food, also benefit digestion. Thus, the command of the Five-Elements Plan, *to eat digestible food*, is almost fulfilled here. To fulfill it entirely, most of the food you eat should be cooked.

People who have a *warm breakfast* consisting of cooked grains, with preserved fruits or cooked vegetables, several days a week will fare the best. A light meat broth with vegetables, or millet with scrambled eggs, also make for a good foundation for the whole morning. Several days of having a breakfast consisting of cooked grains such as millet or polenta, together with stewed fruit, cooked vegetables, aromatic cinnamon, or fresh herbs, will eliminate any ravenous hunger for sweets you may have had. In addition, after several weeks of starting the day this way, if you were overweight you will probably lose weight. The grains can be precooked for two to three days, and the fruits or vegetables cut into small pieces and steamed quickly.

Anyone who has gotten used to eating essentially cooked food, along with salads, fresh herbs, sprouts, or some fresh fruit, will easily forgo eating heavy meals of, say, bread and cold cuts, because they simply don't want to give up their enhanced vitality and overall sense of well-being. The quality and digestibility of various foods, as well as the advantages and disadvantages of common preparation methods, will be discussed in greater detail in the following chapters.

The Thermal Effects of Foods

@

Traditional Chinese dietetics classifies foods into categories according to their thermal, or temperature, effect. There are *hot, warm, neutral, refreshing,* and *cold* foods. The precise allocation of various foods is shown in Appendix B.

Foods are warmed up slightly in terms of their thermal effect through cooking. But the more important benefit of cooked food is their *improvement in digestibility.* The same principle holds true for cold water and juices: When diluted with hot water, they can be tolerated much better. In China, people attach great importance to the digestibility of food, so the Chinese eat only very small quantities of uncooked food.

When certain food like broth has to be cooked very long, there is a loss of enzymes, which stimulate digestion. Thus, small amounts of *food containing enzymes,* such as fermented horseradish or soy sauce, are used as a substitute in certain dishes. Having a teaspoon of fermented vinegar or a piece of umeboshi plum, about the size of a penny, after dinner also stimulates digestion, as both contain large quantities of enzymes. Umeboshi plums are very sour and salty, and are available at health-food stores. When added to dishes at the very end of the cooking process, soy sauce has the same effect. Good-quality brands of soy sauce are Shoyu and Tamari.

The following criteria for healthy nutrition sheds light on the thermal effect of foods:

❀ A large content of water indicates a cooling influence. Vegetables that are forced to grow quickly with a lot of fertilizer contain more water and are more cooling than organically grown vegetables, and less tasty.

❀ Generally, fruits are harvested before they have fully ripened and sweetened, so that they do not go bad as quickly. The artificial process of having them ripen later cannot be compared with the ripening process that takes place in nature. Fruits that have not completely ripened before being picked are much more cooling and less digestible. This is why many people who, on the recommendation of certain diets, eat only fruit for breakfast suffer from a yang deficiency.

❀ Another important consideration has to do with where the fruits and the vegetables that we eat are grown. Fruits grown in countries with a warm climate are generally more cooling than fruits grown in a cold climate, offering the people living there a counterbalance to the heat. On the other hand, people who live in the temperate parts of the United States and Central Europe, for example, tend to eat a lot of tropical fruit, even in the winter, and for them this produces internal coldness. Especially the Middle Burner is cooled and weakened. The spleen and the stomach are unable to extract sufficient qi from the food, causing at first a qi deficiency and as a consequence a yang deficiency, which can lead to cold illnesses. Ironically, this is exactly what people tried to avoid by eating tropical fruits, because of their high content of vitamin C. Above all, our chances of coming down with a head cold depend on whether or not the body has sufficient qi and warmth to fight off the external cold. In summary, *the foods we need grow exactly in the region where we live.* For example, winter vegetables, such as leeks and cabbage, which are still harvested after the first snow in some places, are warming and thus balance the external cold influence.

The criteria above, much of it well accepted now in the West, are important, centuries-old principles of Chinese dietetics. Intuition, observation, experience, and the understanding of cosmic laws, to which human beings and the rest of nature are subjected, made it possible for Chinese healers to understand the thermal effects of foods and their influence on each of the internal organs. The work begun by these ancient healers has continued in the West as well as the East, so many of the foods that are common today in the United States and Europe have been classified according to their thermal nature.

How Do the Different Thermal Effects of Foods Influence the Organism?

@

Hot Foods Protect Us from Coldness

Hot foods, like lamb, garlic, pepper, nutmeg, and chili, and hot beverages, such as hot spicy wine and high-proof alcohol, have a heating, yang-enhancing effect on the body. Their main task is to prevent a deficiency of yang, meaning a state of coldness. As long as the organs have enough warmth, they can function and the qi will flow. If there is a loss of warmth due to cold weather or cold food, the ability of the organs to function decreases and the qi stagnates. Therefore, hot foods are used mainly in the cold season, when the body needs to be protected from the cold weather and there is a greater chance of catching a head cold.

When you feel a head cold coming on, sometimes a glass of hot spicy wine before bed can work wonders by the next morning. The earlier you use the remedy, the better the results. If you get caught in a downpour while riding your bike, for example, it's best not to even wait until the first symptoms appear, but to drink a cup of Indian spice tea or a glass of hot spicy wine as soon as you get home. But it's not a good idea to drink alcohol before going out in cold weather, as the pungent taste opens up the pores and the cold can penetrate even more.

If we consume too much hot food, the body very quickly reaches a yang state, where there is the danger of the fluids drying out and of a deficiency of yin developing. It's not unusual for an excess of yang to occur if you have inherited a yang constitution and have a preference for Indian food, which is typically very hot and spicy and therefore heating. Drinking several cups of coffee every day, on a regular basis, can also bring about an excess of yang; drinking high-proof alcohol regularly has the same effect.

53

How Do the Different Thermal Effects of Food Influence the Organism?

Warm Foods Increase Activity

Everything that holds true for hot foods, is, in a more moderate way, also valid for warm foods, like leeks, onions, fresh ginger, coriander, marjoram, coffee, and red wine. Therefore, in cold weather and during the cold season, warm foods should be consumed in higher quantities.

Movement produces warmth and facilitates the excretion of toxins. People who sit a great deal and who are frequently cold thus enhance their overall well-being and their organs' ability to function when they eat more warming foods and cooked meals.

Vegetable soups and meat broths that have simmered for a long time are a great remedy for getting rid of internal coldness. Because they are so digestible, soups are especially suitable for the lunch break at work. By nature, women have less qi and warmth than men, and are higher in fluids and blood. That's the reason why women tend to be cold more often. Because men are lower in fluids, and have more qi and warmth instead, they tend to suffer from heat or a lack of yin. Interestingly, women are often seen in restaurants eating a salad, while men are enjoying a steak. Knowing their proclivities, wouldn't it be better the other way around?

You should be aware that small amounts of warming food eaten regularly is helpful, but too much warming food like red meat, pungent spices, coffee, and red wine may lead to inner tension, hyperactivity, restlessness, emotionality, and irritability—all signs of an excess of yang.

Neutral Foods Supply Qi

Neutral foods—especially those with a sweet or mild taste like grains, starchy vegetables, beef, and legumes—build up qi and have a balancing effect on the organs. A deficiency or an excess of qi and fluids is eliminated or avoided completely when cooked grain is a mainstay of one's basic diet. Most of the substances that the body needs are contained in grains. Therefore, we can live healthily without deficiencies on very simple meals containing grains, vegetables, some fresh herbs, and legumes, which are the essential protein suppliers in a vegetarian diet, or once in a while adding such common sources of protein as meat, fish, and eggs. I believe that food high in protein should be eaten often, perhaps three to five times a week, but in very small quantities.

Grains

All grains are classified as "neutral," which means balanced, because they reflect the "golden mean": They strengthen the yin and yang roots equally, building up qi as well as fluids. But some grains have an additional special effect of particularly building up either yin or qi. Those grains classified as "refreshing" especially build up yin, and those classified as "warming" chiefly strengthen qi and yang. Wheat, for example, builds up qi, but it also has the extra capability of cooling heat, notably in the heart. Thus, wheat is classified as "refreshing" and should not be consumed in high amounts when there is a deficiency of yang.

55

*How Do the
Different
Thermal
Effects of
Food
Influence the
Organism?*

The classification of grains, in regard to taste, is also complex. As all grains have a sweet-mild taste, they are allocated to the *earth element*, the sweet taste, in Chinese dietetics. According to TCM, there are three main factors that characterize food: their thermal effect, their taste, and their special energetic effect on the internal organs from another element. Food can be sour, bitter, sweet, pungent, or salty. *Each taste corresponds to one of the five elements: Sour food corresponds to wood, bitter food to fire, sweet food to earth, pungent food to metal, and salty food to water.*

Even though they are sweet in taste, which indicates their effect on the organs from the earth element, certain grains have a special energetic or therapeutic effect on the organs from another element. Thus, for the sake of clarity, they are listed where they have their special effect. For example, like all grains, rice is considered mild-sweet. It builds up the qi of the spleen, but has in addition a strengthening effect on the lungs and the large intestine from the *metal element*. Therefore, it is listed with the pungent foods that belong to the metal element.

A Kernel of Grain Is a Small Miracle

Like any seed, a kernel of grain contains the energetic potential of the whole plant. Kernels of grain thousands of years old found in graves have even germinated after having been planted. However, grain will not germinate if you water it with cold water heated before in a microwave.

Several outstanding characteristics are combined in grains. They contain a form of qi that supplies all the internal organs in a well-balanced manner; this is very harmonizing for the person as a whole. The healthy organism digests cooked grain slowly and without much effort. Therefore, it sustains the body for a long time and satisfies many bodily needs. After eating a meal containing cooked whole grain, people normally do not get hungry for several hours, which is also very economical; in addition, they will hardly ever crave sweets or coffee anymore, which is very good for the nerves and for staying slim.

Bread can be considered the first "fast food." Bread was eaten traditionally in combination with cooked food, but for a long time, because of our hectic lifestyles, much cooked food has been replaced with sandwiches. The way bread is eaten today has all the disadvantages of fast food, even if the bread is of the best quality. By no means is a sandwich a substitute for a filling, highly digestible, and qi-strengthening cooked meal. Thus, if you are a passionate bread-eater, and especially if you want to lose weight, I recommend a change in eating habits. Instead of eating bread, try eating more cooked meals for at least two weeks.

It's not the bread by itself that is the entire problem, but also the sweet, salty, and fatty coating, which causes the qi of digestion to weaken and leads to a buildup of dampness in the body. Another reason for the accumulation of dampness when we eat a lot of bread stems from the preference today for eating fresh bread. In the past, people knew that fresh bread causes flatulence and is hard to digest. Bread that is a couple of days old and dry on the inside, as opposed to being moist and sticky, is digested much more easily.

It's a phenomenon of recent times to grab a slice of toast and a cup of coffee for breakfast while running out the door. On the other hand, cooked whole grains, such as wheat, millet, or polenta, prepared with fruits and nuts or with some vegetables, herbs, butter, or egg, are rejuvenating and will appease your hunger until you are ready for lunch.

57

How Do the

Different

Thermal

Effects of

Food

Influence the

Organism?

A warm breakfast works wonders for people who are overweight and who crave sweets. I can testify to this from my many years of experience as a nutritional counselor. It is also a common occurrence that children's grades improve when children start the day with a substantial cooked breakfast. And having tried mildly spicy chicken soup with vegetables and grains in the morning, many an entire family won't do without it. As strange as this may seem for breakfast, it is a great way to refuel your energy for the day, and it is the daily breakfast of billions of people all over Asia.

Grain Calms the Mind

In America, the Indian tribes who had settled in one place and whose basic nutrition was grain were more peaceful than the nomadic tribes who lived for the most part on meat. In India, the majority of the population living in the countryside are vegetarian, whereas the city people tend to eat meat, in order to be able to withstand the daily stresses of a city.

Grains and vegetables have the special ability, when they are cooked, to excrete toxins from the body. A lack of movement, cooling nutrition, and emotional frustration all lead to a deficiency of qi and to qi stagnation. In such cases, food is not digested completely and deposits are converted into toxins. Therefore, especially people who are sedentary should eat a lot of grain, combined with aromatic spices and herbs, in order to prevent this process from occurring. When the organs are nourished in a balanced manner and the qi flows harmoniously, the mind is at peace; this provides an ideal basis for meditating, for doing the slow, flowing movements of tai chi and qigong, or engaging in creative pursuits.

Meat

Beef is another "neutral" food. It is an important source for vitality and the ability to concentrate, because it builds up qi and blood. Today, one of the most widely held half-truths is that meat is bad for us. However, should you get to eat a small piece of eatable meat after some weeks of trekking in the Himalayas, for example, you have the unique opportunity to see for yourself how enormously nourishing meat is. And many people who move to countries where hygienic food is a scarce commodity and they are forced to do without meat soon miss it. Yet, like everything that can be said regarding nutrition, it all depends on the individual. A small percentage of the world's population has such a well-functioning metabolism that their bodies utilize nearly all food components—these people can practically live on air. For most of us, however, eating small amounts of high-quality meat, from naturally raised animals, is good for our health and vitality. The bad reputation that meat has gained is probably due to poor-quality meats and to the disreputable way animals are often raised; many people demonstrate against the conditions animals are subjected to rather than the eating of meat.

From a health perspective, it's important to counteract the various signs of a lack of vitality, such as problems with concentration, fatigue, feeling cold, and a decrease in libido. If you want to dedicate yourself with all your strength to your life and work, just 2 tablespoons of meat per meal three or four times a week can be sufficient. Should you want to consume even less meat, every now and then replace it with some fresh fish or eggs.

Pork is another "neutral" meat that builds up qi. Additionally, it nourishes yin. But when eaten in large quantities and regularly, especially in the form of salty sausage, it will result in water retention in the body and the accumulation of phlegm. This in turn can eventually lead to lethargy, dullness, lack of focus, and being overweight. This condition, sometimes called the "flock-of-sheep syndrome," which is also brought on by consuming large quantities of sweets, seems to be the main cause for that passive habit of spending one's leisure time in front of the TV. It's been said that, thousands of years ago, a Chinese king took advantage of this lethargy-causing effect of pork by allowing his people to eat only this kind of meat in order to control them better.

It's not meat itself that is bad for us, but often the quality, the large quantities consumed, and its unbalanced preparation. As is the case with all foods high in protein, meat is hard to digest. Therefore, it should be prepared in a way that makes it digested more easily. Meat that has been frozen is especially hard to digest, and thus very likely to create the most harmful toxins in the body. These effects are even worsened when the meat is thawed or cooked in a microwave oven. When fried meat is eaten frequently, the organism heats up. Eating hard-to-digest, fried meat often leads to an excess of yang and to deposits of toxins. Both conditions make it more likely that serious illnesses like cancer and heart ailments will develop, and they form the basis for hyperacidity, which tends to foster chronic diseases.

People who are prone to heat symptoms and hyperactivity and experience hot sensations in the body should restrict their consumption of meat. On the other hand, meals containing a small amount of meat are a cure for people who get cold easily and are frequently tired. In addition, the deposits of toxins are avoided for the most part when meat is cooked with vegetables and especially with fresh ginger.

Sausage usually has too much salt, but beyond that it's often difficult to tell what it contains. However, if you can't resist having sausage with your eggs, it is crucial that it be of good quality and eaten only in small amounts. But anyone who exchanges a sandwich of cold cuts for a cheese sandwich is not doing him- or herself a favor. The cooling and phlegm-producing effects of too much cheese result more quickly in the flock-of-sheep syndrome—that is, in a deficiency of qi, water retention, and being overweight—than too much pork does.

There are many good reasons, both ethical and economical, to forgo meat; in addition, a vegetarian diet is basically healthier than a diet with a lot of meat, as meat is difficult to digest and produces deposits of toxins. However, anyone who wants to eat a vegetarian diet and lives in a cold climate must do some cooking regularly to avoid the deficiencies of qi and blood, which often occur in vegetarians. For most of the vegetarians I see in my practice, I can't avoid recommending three cooked meals a day in order to get rid of the symptoms of a yang deficiency, including frequent urination, urination during the night, cold feet, and back pain.

Cooked food, including grains and neutral vegetables like white cabbage and carrots, is necessary for supplying the body with sufficient qi and warmth and for producing blood. Meat broths and meals containing small quantities of meat are a suitable therapeutic remedy for building up qi and blood noticeably and quickly when there are deficiencies in these areas. For meat to fulfill this purpose, however, it must come from animals raised appropriately. In addition, the meat should not have been frozen, because then it is hard to digest and it does more damage than good.

61

How Do the
Different
Thermal
Effects of
Food
Influence the
Organism?

Legumes

You will get the best results if you eat, on a regular basis, along with grains and vegetables, small quantities of legumes. Lentils, peas, and beans are high-quality protein suppliers, and they are eaten daily by those groups in the population who are forced to be vegetarians—that is, primarily by people living in poor, hot countries, like India.

In order for legumes to be digested more easily, it is recommended to prepare them with fresh ginger, caraway, or other spices and herbs that foster digestion. In addition, it isn't a good idea to use the water in which they were soaking for cooking, because it contains precisely those substances that cause flatulence. Salt and a small amount of vinegar are added only at the end of the cooking process. If you add salt at the beginning, the legumes do not become soft. Also, to make them more digestible, and at the same time to supply the body with lots of minerals, legumes can be cooked together with a small amount of seaweed like wakame, kombu, or hijiki, available at health-food stores.

Refreshing Foods Increase the Buildup of Blood

The body builds up blood and fluids from "refreshing" foods. In order for this to happen, the responsible organs, the spleen and the kidneys, need sufficient qi. Thus, if there is a deficiency of blood and fluids, it is important, above all, to build up qi with the help of neutral and warm foods, while building up fluids with the help of refreshing foods. Most vegetables and fruits and some salads fall into the "refreshing" category. Everything that is green from the world of plants is excellent for building up blood. It is best to increase the amount of green, leafy salads and herbs in the summer and spring, and to reduce them to a smaller amount in the fall and winter, when warming food is preferred.

Only a small portion of our meals should consist of uncooked food, in the form of raw vegetables, fresh fruits, and salads. This may come as a surprise to you, as uncooked food is higher in vitamins than cooked food and is thus often praised highly. But it's been less than a hundred years since vitamins were discovered. And until a few decades ago, the few vegetables that enriched the menu were usually overcooked, and fruits and salads were served only when they were in season. So, perhaps our tendency to overvalue everything that is new and condemn everything that is old has shaped our view when it comes to this matter.

In England, in the year 1917, 41 percent of the men in their prime were unfit for military service because they were malnourished. In Vienna in 1919, most of the babies and young children suffered from scurvy or rickets, caused from a lack of vitamins. Thus, the discovery of vitamins was a blessing that healed many people and prevented them from dying at a young age.

Yet cautious scientists concede that even today not all facets of nutrition are understood. Science knows even less about the holistic effect of individual foods and their collaboration. Although the supermarkets today are fully stocked with fresh fruits and vegetables, even in the dead of winter, the problem concerning a lack of vitamins still seems to persist with certain individuals. As already mentioned, there are a variety of reasons for this: Pesticides, overexploited soil, and overcultivation all contribute to the fact that fruits and vegetables nowadays comprise only a fraction of the nutrients they contained sixty years ago. But there is another reason for a lack of vitamins today: More than 90 percent of the food eaten in the United States is "packed," which means that its ingredients are denatured through industrial production. What this means is that the naturally contained vitamins are disturbed in the process and are substituted with synthetic vitamins, even though they lack all the healthful effects described on the package.

Traditional Chinese medicine, however, offers another viewpoint. Because many people tend to consume uncooked food, tropical fruits, milk products, and sweets, as well as fast food, they suffer from a deficiency of qi in the Middle Burner, the part of the body that is mainly responsible for the gaining of postnatal qi. The result is that a major part of the vital substances in food cannot be utilized and is excreted instead.

The many unbalanced fad diets, which propagate one approach for everybody and are so popular today, are also to blame. Some of these diets emphasize eating an abundance of raw fruits and vegetables over cooked foods, which can actually make us sick. This holds true especially for women and especially in the winter. Limited amounts of uncooked food are good for people who work hard physically or are otherwise especially active, like competitive athletes and people with an excess of yang that expresses itself through a fiery temperament and hyperactivity. *In all other people, but particularly in those who sit a great deal and do a lot of brainwork, large quantities of uncooked food lead to a deficiency of qi, internal coldness, weakened immunity, poor concentration, digestive problems, depression, and low libido.*

The effects of improper nutrition are most noticeable in babies and small children. For instance, infants who are fed bananas when they are still lying in their cradles have problems with digestion, and a pale complexion and rings under the eyes can already be seen in the smallest of children. When they are of school age, concentration disorders, a deficiency of qi, proneness to head colds, and unsatisfactory achievement in school are the consequences. If you feed your children cooked multigrain cereal and hot soups instead of tropical fruits and milk products, you won't have to pay for a tutor. Investing time into the preparation of meals is definitely worthwhile.

The Chinese have this saying: "The human being distinguishes himself from the animal through his intellect and through the fact that he cooks his meals. With the fire used in cooking, the intellectual and spiritual fire of the human being is kindled."

Cooking

Especially for refreshing foods—that is, most vegetables and fruit—which are usually eaten raw nowadays, cooking plays an important, balancing role. Unfortunately, eating hot cereal with stewed fruit has gone out of fashion and many children now know tomato sauce only from the ketchup bottle. But the cooking process is crucial, because it prepares food in such a way that it can be digested easily by the body.

65

How Do the
Different
Thermal
Effects of
Food
Influence the
Organism?

The expenditure of qi for the digestion of cooked food is much lower than that for uncooked food. In addition, the body must first warm up food that is uncooked, which also uses up qi. An old proverb says: "Soups make fat." Why? Because soups warm up the stomach so comfortably, causing digestion to work so well, that we can eat much more afterward. In contrast to many animals, the digestive tract of most people can digest a fraction of the vegetables and fruits that are eaten uncooked. The remainder is excreted, without any vitamins or nutrients having been extracted. It is different with cooked food, even if it has been cooked for a short time. The cooked food can be utilized better energetically, and the nutrients reach the body. This is also the case when it is eaten later cold.

In summary, it can be said that cooked refreshing foods like baked apples and stewed tomatoes build up a lot more fluids in the body than refreshing foods like fruits, vegetables, and salads that are eaten uncooked and than fruit and vegetable juices. Fresh herbs and leafy salads made of chicory, endive, and radicchio are much more nourishing and digestible when they are eaten in combination with cooked food, as opposed to raw tomatoes and cucumber, which should enrich meals only in small quantities because they are colder in their thermal effect.

Cold Foods Protect Us from Heat

Many tropical fruits and herbal teas, as well as tomatoes, cucumber, yogurt, seaweed, mineral water, and salt fall into in the "cold" category. Consuming a small quantity of cold foods in meals prevents the development of too much heat, or a yang excess, in the body. The cold foods offer a counterbalance to hot weather, especially in the summer and in hot countries. Otherwise, what was said for refreshing food holds true for cold food, except that the cooling effect of cold food occurs faster and penetrates deeper into the body. Particularly in the summer, a qi weakness of the digestive tract and of the Middle Burner frequently develop when people consume too much cold food, ice cream, and ice-cold beverages. As a result, the kidneys in the Lower Burner are increasingly forced to supply warmth and qi. Eventually, this leads to a yang deficiency of the kidneys and a state of internal coldness, with such symptoms as lack of performance ability, fatigue, and low libido.

Of course, people have more of a need for refreshing and cold foods in the summer, when many people restrict their diet to salads, uncooked food, fruits, fruit juices, frozen yogurt, and ice cream. In addition, water and other beverages are often drunk ice-cold. This unbalanced diet leads, particularly if there is already a latent lack of qi, to the conditions described above. In order to avoid this, it is important to consume cold foods carefully even in the summer.

In general, it's best to forgo ice-cold drinks, because they cause even in a healthy stomach a cold shock, as the discrepancy between one's body temperature and the cold drink is too great. In hot countries, people drink hot beverages with a cooling thermal effect, such as peppermint tea or green tea. This way, the body is refreshed without cooling down too drastically. Being overweight can often be traced back to a qi weakness of the Middle Burner, caused by the widespread consumption of ice-cold beverages.

Many herbal teas are classified as "cold." Even though the herbs are conducive to health, this fact cannot be concealed. In addition, herbal teas are medicinal, but the opposite effect occurs when they are used incorrectly or for too long. This is true for chamomile tea, peppermint tea, lady's mantle tea, and even for fruit teas. But when used in proper quantities, based on knowledge of their effects, herbal teas are helpful and don't do any damage.

Drinking Water

Hot water, perhaps with some honey or sugar, a drop of vinegar or lemon, or simply "à la nature," is the ideal beverage. I was astonished when I first came upon this healthy way of drinking water, visiting a Tibetan monk. After I tried it myself, it seemed completely natural. Cold water falls into the "cold" category, especially when it contains too many minerals and sodium. By preparing tea with warming spices like star anise, cinnamon, and ginger, or by simply heating water, the cooling effect is balanced. By the way, this also works with other beverages. When you are cold and prefer a hot drink, try heating up apple juice or grape juice for a change. It tastes delicious, and your belly will feel nice and warm.

The Correct Selection
of Foods

According to the Chinese professor Leung Kok Yuen, who is advanced in age and now lives in Canada, a healthy diet consists of 70 percent grains, 15 percent cooked vegetables, 5 percent uncooked food, 5 percent meat or fish, and 5 percent milk products and other miscellaneous foods.

Don't worry—I am not trying to convince you to eat this way. Yet if you are basically healthy and want to try this diet for a few days a month, and then grow to like it, I can only congratulate you. Not only will you be changing your general eating habits step-by-step in the direction of a more healthy diet, but you will also in the long run have an above-average metabolism, as well as almost certainly good overall health, an inner calmness, and a long life. I also mention this diet so that you will know how people who take care of their health according to the principles of TCM balance the different aspects of their nutrition, as well as understand why they seem generally so calm and even-tempered.

But you should not force yourself to eat this way or follow any other nutritional regime. Nutritional habits evolve for us on an individual basis by consciously paying attention to how a certain food we introduce into our diet agrees with us. In order to do this, it's necessary to try out the food for some time and become adept at its methods of preparation. If you, for example, have cooked with heavy cream frequently until now and want to get away from that, say, by using more herbs and spices, you'll need to be creative and practice a little.

It is not a matter of forcing yourself to eliminate everything from your diet that you have recognized as being unwholesome. On the contrary, by starting to make use of the abundance of foods and preparation methods suggested here, many unwholesome habits and exaggerated cravings will disappear on their own. Anyone who uses too much force easily falls into the power of some other unhealthy extreme.

Nutrition must fit like a well-cut suit. It must be flexible and adaptable to personal taste; then it will become a friend for life. To the degree that we change and go through different life phases, our dietary habits also change. By saying this, I do not mean that we should try out one diet after another; I mean just the opposite—that it's important to find a basis at some point in life and to see what positive effects certain foods have or what damage they can do. When this information has become part of your life, it is quite simple to choose the foods most suitable for yourself at any given time. Chinese dietetics is a good friend. It will assist you all your life, in good times and in bad, and it will help you to master difficult phases. As a true friend, however, it will not always approve of everything you do, and thus will help you give up cherished but bad habits and discover something new.

Recently I met an old girlfriend with whom I had shared an apartment several years ago. The last time I saw her, six years ago, she was involved in Chinese dietetics and following a grain diet. She was in the process of just getting rid of the last few pounds and of harmonizing her system. In the meantime, she had graduated from college and was successful in her job, and now she stood before me lean and happy. Casually she told me that she was often asked how she had succeeded in remaining so slim, having tried various diets in the past with less success. Now she was telling everybody that they should eat whatever they wanted at the moment, as that was what she did herself.

Astonished, I asked her if she had given up following the guidelines of Chinese dietetics, which had helped her so much, and she became momentarily lost in thought. "No," she responded, "I haven't stopped following them, only I had completely forgotten, because Chinese dietetics has become such a natural part of my life. The things I like are exactly those things that are good for me, so I don't think about it. And once or twice a month I eat ice cream or chocolate, but I simply don't crave them anymore."

In essence, a holistic, balanced nutritional system creates the basis for an unrestricted, independent way of eating. *When the body finally gets what it truly needs, ravenous hunger and strong cravings for sweets, coffee, and alcohol occur less and less.* But even in cases where there is a real problem with addiction, nutrition can also be a great support. However, it will not suffice as the only measure to overcome the addiction, because the damage of the qi and of the fluids has already progressed too far. Within the scope of TCM, acupuncture and herbal therapy will then be used, along with psychotherapy.

The freedom of human beings consists of being able to change with the help of our will and discipline to the degree that we deem right. The mind should dominate the body, and not vice versa. I do not detect any freedom when someone feels compelled to eat a bar of chocolate every day. But exactly how should we deal with strong cravings? It is difficult and most of the time not successful in the long run to prohibit the satisfaction of cravings, because the cause of the craving is still there. It is indeed more helpful to know that ravenous hunger for sweets is a symptom of a qi deficiency of the spleen, which tries in this way to get the taste that will heal it. But the spleen is not saying, "I want chocolate." That is the person's interpretation. According to Chinese dietetics, what the spleen is actually saying is "I want a sweet, warm breakfast, sweet millet, sweet carrots, and sweet beef, in order to build up my qi." I believe that this interpretation is closer to the truth. Try it out for yourself.

It is easier to achieve a healthy mental state with balanced nutrition as a basis. The strengthening of the Middle Burner, which transforms food and stabilizes us, also gives us more distance from emotions, needs, desires, and extreme cravings. Thus, it becomes easier over time to decide freely, I will give in to this, or I can easily forgo that, because I have often experienced that it is not good for me.

Combining Foods according to Their Thermal Effects

There are two areas where Chinese dietetics is applied: daily nutrition for prevention and therapeutic dietetics for treatment. *Therapeutic dietetics* is made use of purposively when an illness has been determined on the basis of a diagnosis according to the principles of TCM. In this case, doctors and nonmedical practitioners prescribe a therapeutic diet based on Chinese dietetics, along with acupuncture and/or herbal therapy. In China, doctors of TCM are astonished when they hear that there are healers in the United States and Europe who practice acupuncture but don't know anything about herbal therapy or dietetics. It is unimaginable for Chinese doctors not to exhaust the different possibilities. The primary aim of *daily nutrition* based on Chinese dietetics is to ensure that illnesses do not develop in the first place. In addition, its purpose is to heal slight imbalances and simple ailments.

People often ask me, "How should I cook at home? All of us have different constitutions, and I can't cook a different meal for everybody." The answer is very simple: Cook in a balanced manner when it comes to the thermal effects of foods, and choose ingredients according to the season; then it will fit everyone's needs. Of course, the five flavors play a role in combining foods, but they will be addressed later.

Concerning the thermal effect of foods, it is especially important that the biggest part of a meal consist of neutral foods and refreshing and warm vegetables. Cold and hot foods should always be used carefully and in small quantities. Stressing the "golden mean" is a guarantee that the organism will balance itself sooner or later. Even though potatoes are neutral, grain has more of a harmonizing, qi-enhancing effect, so they should be regarded like vegetables, which, strictly speaking, they are. Neutral, warm, and refreshing foods create the balanced basis of a meal; hot and cold foods are meant for garnishing. Also during the hot time of the year, it's best not to eat too much cold food. Especially in the summer, the qi is more at the surface of the body, and the inside, chiefly the stomach and the spleen, is particularly susceptible to becoming quite cool.

73

Combining
Foods
according to
Their
Thermal
Effects

Refreshing food is eaten more in the spring and summer, warm food in the fall and winter. Fresh herbs, green leafy salads, sprouts, and fruits in small quantities enrich the menu in every season, but should be used more in the summer and less in the winter.

As mentioned, sandwiches, even when whole-grain bread is used, do not have the same effects as meals with cooked grains, which are more nourishing, sustaining, and warming, are digested better, and supply more qi. People who are overweight without heat symptoms (with a tendency to be rather cold) can reduce their weight dramatically when they eat warm meals three times a day consisting of primarily grain with vegetables and sometimes a little meat. Cold cuts, sausage, cheese, nuts, and marmalade on bread contain a lot of fat, which is not the case with cooked meals or at least not necessary.

If you are not familiar with cooking whole grains, let me give you some advice. First of all, grains such as brown rice or millet are easy to cook, and they are important for our health. If occasionally white flour or spaghetti is part of a meal, it is an enjoyment that you should allow yourself with a good conscience. But should you succeed in incorporating three or four whole-grain meals per week into your menu, you are well on your way.

If you don't like the taste of grain, I ask you to consider how you would like potatoes or spaghetti without any kind of garnishing, spices, or sauce. Probably not at all! That's not true for grain. Brown rice, for example, with a little sea salt and organic butter can be a simple, tasty in-between meal. It is also good to eat when it's merely a matter of appeasing hunger, without especially stressing the body, or if you want to lose weight. And brown rice doesn't take much time to cook. Of course, if the rice is too soft or if the core inside is still uncooked, it will not taste good. If you add garnishing, sauces, herbs, and spices, naturally brown rice will taste even better.

Try the following recipe: Mix champignons, cut in slices, some olive oil, and some grated Parmesan cheese into freshly cooked brown rice. Add a little salt, season with lemon juice, and stir. As an option, you can sprinkle some parsley and tiny pieces of red pepper on top. Then serve immediately. I assure you, this risotto tastes delicious, and it looks very nice!

74

Combining

Foods

according to

Their

Thermal

Effects

Increasing the Yang or the Yin of Food

@

In Chinese dietetics, there are different methods of preparation that increase or balance the thermal effects of foods. In other words, depending on how food is prepared, its yang or yin can be increased. When we want to enlarge the yang of a refreshing food, for example, it's a matter of balancing the refreshing effect of the food through cooking or the use of warming spices. With warm foods, it's a matter of supporting the initial warming effect of the food. Increasing the yin works the other way around. By means of the cooking technique or the use of refreshing or cold ingredients, a warm food is counterbalanced with more yin or the cooling influence of a food is expanded further.

Increasing Yang

Barbecuing, smoking, browning, frying, baking, long simmering in liquid (as with soups), and cooking with alcohol, as well as using hot and warming spices, are all cooking methods that build yang.

Barbecuing produces the most heat in food, because the food has direct contact with the fire or the heat source. Especially meat, when barbecued, receives a strong heating effect that can cause an excess of yang in the area of the stomach. In Italy, the Health Department in Arezzo, Tuscany, came to realize a connection between the frequent barbecuing of meat and the development of stomach cancer. During the long hot summer, people there barbecue their meals daily outside. These meals consist almost exclusively of meat and fried potatoes. Vegetables and salad are eaten only in the smallest quantities. In addition, the wine of this area contains a lot of tannic acid. It's believed that the combination of the barbecued meat and the tannic acid from the wine causes the stomach cancer that is so prevalent in this region. Eating meat in large quantities causes chronic hyperacidity and toxic deposits in the body. When meat is barbecued, because of its direct contact with the heat, and through the smoke that develops when the dripping fat burns in the fire, these deposits are especially toxic. They then accumulate in the body. Traditional Chinese medicine considers these toxic deposits a cause for the development of cancer. When you barbecue anything, or toast bread for that matter, it is important to remove everything that is burnt black, because the charred remains are toxic. Therefore, I advise you to consider barbecuing a luxury that you enjoy only rarely.

Smoking has somewhat less of a heating effect than barbecuing. In addition, the food does not come in direct contact with the fire. Nevertheless, I advise against eating smoked food on a regular basis, as it is also always very salty. Smoked fish, especially salmon, strengthens and warms the kidneys. In the winter, it's helpful to take advantage of this effect from time to time. Yet using bred salmon is extremely questionable. The fish live in very tight spaces, and large quantities of antibiotics and pesticides are used, which eventually end up in the fish. Pregnant women and women who are breastfeeding are advised today by various authorities against eating bred salmon.

Browning meat in a frying pan with fat has an effect

that is similar to that of barbecuing meat, as the food is exposed to strong heat. Especially people who are prone to internal heat should eat blackened or browned steaks as rarely as possible.

Gentle, slow simmering in fat at moderate heat balances the cooling effect of vegetables. Vegetable oils are especially recommended for frying. But many people like to fry with butter because of its taste. It's no problem using butter from time to time as long as you digest it easily without feeling too full. However, you should know that butter, like meat, produces toxic residues and obstructs digestion, particularly in the gallbladder, when it is heated too much. If it's important for you to use butter when frying, the butter should be organic and only heated to such a degree that it doesn't turn brown. It would be even better to add the butter just at the end of the cooking process. The vegetable oils widely used in cooking today are safflower, corn, cottonseed, soybean, and sunflower.

Baking in the oven is a sensible way to balance the cooling effect of vegetables and fruits, and to enhance their digestibility. This is certainly nothing new, as the apple cake is probably as old as the stove. Bodily fluids are built up better with heated fruits, because an overcooling of the digestive organs is avoided. Vegetarians in particular should make use of this warmth-increasing cooking method, because they often develop too little bodily warmth, especially in the winter. When, for example, tomatoes are baked with mozzarella cheese, the meal is less cooling than it is uncooked and much more digestible. Steaming tomatoes, in the preparation of real tomato sauce, is an example of how people who cook Mediterranean style, and especially Italians, regularly take care of the support of their bodily fluids. The tomato sauce from the ketchup jar and bought tomato paste, of course, are no substitute for this.

Simmering soups for a long time is a very gentle, but effective way to nourish the body and build yang. Sometimes meat broths and vegetable soups are cooked for days in China when internal cold needs to be eliminated or it's necessary to build up qi—for example, when recuperating from a long illness or, for new mothers, after giving birth. In gastronomy, the meat bones of a strong and robust soup must be cooked 10 to 15 hours. With this method of food preparation, it is not a matter of nutrition or vitamins, because after several hours of cooking the vitamins of course have been boiled away. It is rather a matter of increasing the warming yang in the food as much as possible through the heat of the cooking.

In the Middle Ages, in the homes in Central and Northern Europe, it was a widespread practice to have large pots permanently hanging in the kitchen above the fireplace. Each day everything that the house, the stable, and the garden had to offer was put into the constantly simmering pot; the fire was never extinguished. This hearty soup was the main source of nutrition for the people. Today's stews are a remnant of this tradition.

Stews, with or without meat, are an excellent source of warmth and qi in the winter. The longer bones and meat are cooked, the more the yang is increased. But when it comes to cooking a vegetable stew, I would discourage you from cooking it too long, because vegetables that are overcooked lose their high nutritive value and the yang-increasing effect can be achieved instead with warm or hot spices and herbs.

Spices not only enhance the flavor of food but also have a strong energetic, or thermal, effect. Pepper, chili, and curry, for example, are hot. Paprika, nutmeg, clove, coriander, caraway seeds, and cinnamon are warm, as are fresh herbs like basil, chive, oregano, thyme, and rosemary. These ingredients warm the digestive tract and thus make it easier for the food to produce postnatal qi. In the winter, they are crucial for protection from cold weather.

Many winter vegetables like cabbage, sauerkraut, and legumes are prepared with warming spices such as bay leaves, juniper berries, caraway seeds, and cloves. These dishes require longer cooking than usual, however, to enhance the warming effect. Red cabbage actually tastes better when it is heated up again. The same holds true for most of the stews and winter dishes. Unfortunately, due to the emphasis today on vitamins, heating up food has become taboo. This is a pity, because what can be faster than cooking a pot of red cabbage that is served two or three days in a row with different side dishes?

Most fruits are refreshing, which makes them an important supplier of bodily fluids. However, the majority of people in the industrial countries—especially women, the elderly, and already many children—have weak digestion, making the cooling effect of fresh fruit undesirable. This is why cooking fruit with warming spices as a stew is especially advised.

Simply put some apple slices together with a little water or fruit juice and some cinnamon in a pot, and let it simmer. You can do the same with all kinds of fruit that are sour, like currants, rhubarb, and gooseberries, for example. Sweetened with honey or fruit juice, this dish is ideal for children, and it can easily be made into muesli (a Swiss breakfast cereal of oats, nuts, and fruit) or a sweet soufflé with cooked grains. Cinnamon, clove powder, cardamom, or ginger balance the cooling effect of the fruit, and the body can produce more of its own fluids as a result of the cooking. With fruit like strawberries, peaches, and nectarines, which contain a lot of water, it is sufficient to heat them up briefly. This way, the flavor and the nutritive value are retained.

Often used in Asian dishes, *fresh ginger* is an exotic spice with a very intense flavor. It goes especially well with all kinds of meat, bean sprouts, and tofu. Ginger, as well as all Indian spices, like masala, cumin, and curry, develop their taste best when added directly into the oil heating up in the frying pan. After the spices have heated up briefly, such ingredients as meat, vegetables, or tofu, cut into small pieces, are added. This gentle method of cooking works particularly well with a wok, as it cooks food fast and all ingredients keep their specific flavor. An Oriental-style chicken soup also tastes delicious when it is prepared with a little fresh ginger, Indian spices, and bean sprouts. Fresh ginger can be used in small quantities on a regular basis and, during the cold season, even more frequently. I always have a small supply in the refrigerator, as it is the best remedy for the common cold and food poisoning. When you realize that a cold is coming on, a cup of ginger tea works real wonders. It's also a good remedy when you have eaten an overly rich meal.

Peel a piece of ginger, about the size of two cloves of garlic, cut it into slices, and simmer it about 10 minutes in half a quart, or liter, of water. Pour it into a strainer, and drink the tea at the beginning of a cold or when you feel nauseous. Due to the very pungent taste of this beverage, internal cold is banished and all damaging bacteria in the intestine disappear.

In hot countries, where all food goes bad quickly, many hot spices are used for the same reason. The heat of these pungent spices, however, is not good for people living in hot climates, which is why many Indians and Nepalese are sick. Yet they need the hot spices to protect themselves from the many bacteria.

For trips and for your medicine chest at home, ginger can be preserved in alcohol. Peel a piece of ginger, cut it into slices, and leave it in half a quart, or liter, of vodka for a week. Then strain it. On a trip to Asia, I drank a teaspoon of ginger schnapps after every meal the first few days when my body was especially vulnerable to the unfamiliar bacteria. I'm convinced that saved me from getting sick.

If you are constantly feeling cold or you have cold feet, you can cure yourself by using daily, for one to two weeks, a small amount of ginger in your food, or by drinking a cup of mild ginger tea. Because of its warming and qi-stagnation-combating effect, ginger is among the most important remedies of Chinese pharmacology. For people who suffer from a condition of heat, however, ginger is only advisable in cases of emergency. Ginger powder is not very intense in taste, but it is actually much hotter in its thermal effect than fresh ginger. Therefore, it should be used infrequently and in small amounts, as should chili powder.

Cooking with alcohol is a very tasty and refined method of food preparation that also builds up yang. The higher the percentage of alcohol, the more heating is the effect.

Try the following recipe: Cut poultry into small pieces. Chop a piece of fresh ginger very finely, and mix together. Then place the mixture in a bowl as small as possible, so that the pieces of meat are close together, and pour sake (rice wine) and some soy sauce over it until the meat is covered. It should soak for at least several hours, but preferably overnight. Then take out the meat, let the liquid drip off, and brown it in a frying pan on the burner. Add the marinade it had been soaking in, and let it simmer for a couple more minutes. Finally season it any way you like, possibly with honey, chili, Tabasco sauce, and salt. You can also add cashew nuts, roasted walnuts, or chestnuts. Brown rice or basmati rice, vegetables such as bean sprouts, peppers, and cabbage, and a crisp salad go well with this dish.

Lamb in red wine is a very warming dish for the winter. Cut the lamb into small pieces. Mix it with onion slices, chopped garlic, and rosemary. Pour a dry red wine over it. Let the meat soak from 6 hours up to a couple of days. The longer the meat stays in the marinade, the tarter it will taste. Remove the lamb mixture from the wine, and let the wine drip off. Remove the onion slices, and put them aside. Brown the meat in a frying pan on the burner. Now add the onion slices, which have also been drained well of the liquid, and simmer until all the liquid is gone. Add a little marinade, and let it simmer down. When the meat is done, add the remaining marinade and let everything simmer for a couple more minutes. Add some salt and it's done. If the taste is too tart for you, try serving this dish with cranberry marmalade. Boiled potatoes and a crisp salad are good side dishes. If you don't care for lamb, use beef. Red wine enhances their qi-increasing effect; it also works well with goulash and meat dishes made with paprika and chili.

Eating food cooked with alcohol causes the qi to rise up in the body. This effect is especially desired when the Middle Burner (the spleen and the stomach) or the Upper Burner (the heart and the lungs) suffer from a deficiency of qi, as the qi sinks down in these cases. A sign of this condition is a weakness in digestion with soft stools. Within the parameters of the psyche, depression, sadness, frustration, or resignation can occur. If the lungs are weakened, a hanging posture is frequently seen, and the person often feels exhausted easily when talking, meaning that the voice is weak. The person is also prone to head colds and to low blood pressure. In all these cases, cooking with alcohol helps to enhance vitality, as blockages are dissolved and the qi rises up.

Increasing Yin

When it comes to increasing yin, it is a matter of reducing the warming effect of a food or of enhancing a food's cooling nature. This balancing is best applied to warm meats such as poultry and game, hot meats like lamb, and browned or blackened beef. Intensifying the cooling effect can be desirable for cooling vegetables like cauliflower, cucumber, and zucchini.

The following cooking methods are used for building yin: *blanching, steaming briefly, and cooking with such ingredients as fruit, sprouts, seaweed, fruit juices, and champignons.*

When vegetables and fruits are *blanched,* their refreshing character is preserved. They merely become more digestible by being heated up briefly. Usually, a lot of water is used for this, which is poured out afterward together with many nutrients that have dissolved in it.

Steaming briefly, using a small amount of water, is a much better method: Cut the vegetables into very small pieces, put them in the steamer, and it will take only a couple of minutes until they are done. This way, they preserve their full aroma and almost all their vitamins. This procedure is especially well suited for the morning meal should you want to prepare a mild-tasting, crunchy, digestible vegetable dish with little fat. Carrots, combined with other vegetables, are particularly suitable for this.

Fruits can be briefly stewed, as well, and enhanced with cinnamon, coriander, vanilla, and nuts. At the end, you can add some organic butter, cold-pressed oil, or a nut puree, so that the dish will sustain you longer. Cooking with cold fruit like kiwi brings a refining touch to sliced-poultry dishes and has a balancing effect when heating spices like curry and chili are used. In such cases, it is sufficient to place the fruit, cut into slices, over the dish, and then to serve it immediately. You can do the same with *sprouts* from watercress and alfalfa. Sprouts that were grown from grain or legumes, however, should be cooked briefly with the meat.

Dried *seaweed* like hijiki and wakame are cooked along with soups and stews for some minutes. When dishes are cooked only briefly, the dried seaweed is soaked in hot water for half an hour and then added. Small quantities—about 2 tablespoons of hijiki or a piece of wakame about 6 inches, or 15 centimeters, long—two to three times a week are sufficient to supply the organism with a large variety of minerals and to protect it from a deficiency of yin.

Especially with women during menopause, when the yin decreases rapidly and extensively, seaweed counteracts such unpleasant yin deficiencies as hot flashes and night sweats. In addition, seaweed—when eaten regularly—is known to prevent osteoporosis (bone decalcification). Although it's a widespread belief that milk products are good for this, research has concluded that a high consumption of cheese, milk, and sour-milk products actually expedites the development of osteoporosis. And in China, where no milk products are consumed whatsoever, osteoporosis after menopause is not the common occurrence that it is elsewhere. So, all of this should get us thinking.

Essentially, the weakness of the digestive tract and the consumption of too much processed food are responsible for the body's demineralization. Stress is also a mineral thief. Thus, it is increasingly important for women (and men) from age thirty-five on, to strengthen the qi of the Middle Burner and, at the same time, to make sure that the body is supplied with minerals through sufficient sleep and high-quality fluid-building nutrition. Green vegetables, leafy salads, fresh herbs, and especially different types of seaweed contain large quantities of calcium and other minerals that help prevent osteoporosis, night sweats, troubled sleep, and nervousness.

If you are hesitant to cook with seaweed, you can make a seaweed tea: Pour hot water over a tablespoon of hijiki or a 6-inch (15-centimeter) piece of wakame. Wait until the seaweed has soaked sufficiently, and then add some more hot water. Now drink the hot liquid and eat the seaweed, because it contains most of the minerals. If you have any of the above-mentioned ailments, drink the tea three to four times a week in the afternoon or the evening.

Fruit juices such as organic red grape juice, which builds up blood, are suitable for salad dressings or for sauces used with sweet-grain dishes. Semolina or millet, cooked in water, can be enhanced at the end of the cooking process with fruit juice, in order to increase their yin-building effect. But if you cook the fruit juices with the grains, they taste a little sour.

Fruit juices are digested better when they are mixed with hot water. Again and again, I've noticed adults ordering a hot drink—tea or coffee—in a cafe or restaurant, while children are drinking ice-cold fruit juice, even though they might prefer to drink something hot. Unfortunately, there is hardly any choice for them. However, in such cases and also at home, it is possible to dilute the juices, which are too sweet in the first place, with hot water.

Natural, unsweetened or organic apple juice is well suited for building up yin. For children and adults, apple juice is digested better if you fix it this way: Prepare a spice tea by simmering a selection of the following spices 10 to 20 minutes in water: cinnamon-stick, star anise, fennel, ginger, and cardamom. Then add some sugar and as much apple juice as you like. Children love this combination, especially in the winter.

Champignons have, aside from their moistening and cooling effects, another special advantage: They help to make meat and egg dishes more digestible and thus counteract deposits of toxins. Because champignons are domesticated, they do not contain heavy metals and radioactivity like forest mushrooms, so they can be eaten without hesitation. For the Chinese, they are a remedy for long life because of their manifold harmonizing effects. They strengthen the digestive tract, reduce internal heat, harmonize the flow of qi, and calm the mind, all sufficient reasons for using them in our cooking more frequently.

A very tasty, refreshing risotto is prepared as follows: Add champignons, cut into thin slices, a small amount of tomatoes, the green part of green onions or chives, chopped finely, and sesame oil to brown rice that is already cooked. Season with lemon juice and salt and pepper, mix, and serve immediately. This risotto goes well with asparagus, many other vegetables, and meat dishes.

@

These yin- or yang-increasing methods can help you cook with more creativity and purpose. In order to achieve a certain goal—for example, to give a dish a refreshing effect in the summer—you will likely need to use a different cooking technique from what you are accustomed to. Please don't consider this a restriction but rather an invitation to try something new. You will have many pleasant surprises as you abandon your old habits and open up to new foods and different methods of preparation. In addition, you will be assured that you are doing something good for yourself and for others as you learn to cook delicious meals following the principles of Chinese dietetics.

The Golden Mean

The following guidelines, based on the "golden mean" of Taoism and Chinese dietetics, which has to do with practicing moderation and avoiding extremes, will help you develop an overall orientation to balanced, healthy nutrition:

@ Use as often as possible gentle and neutral methods for preparing food. For instance, it's much better to steam vegetables with a little water at a low temperature than frying them in fat over a high heat, as the latter method, among other things, is rough on digestion. If you cut vegetables into small pieces, steam them briefly, and then add some tasty oil like olive oil, sesame oil, pumpkinseed oil, or peanut oil, they will be digested much better than if you fry the vegetables in oil right from the beginning.

@ Cut down on yang-building cooking methods during the hot season. Use less hot spices and more fresh herbs. Enjoy the full flavor of the vegetables and salad greens that grow outside.

@ It's important for vegetarians to absorb enough qi and yang through food during each season. Therefore, my advice to vegetarians is to *cook!* If you already suffer from coldness, it may be necessary to eat cooked food almost exclusively during the winter. It's certainly favorable to bake dishes in the oven more often, regularly using warm and hot spices and herbs. Drinking warming teas made with spices like cinnamon or

Caraway is recommended, as is plain hot water. Cold water, especially mineral water, containing sodium, has a cold effect. In comparison to a cheese sandwich, a can of soup or a cup of instant dehydrated vegetable soup to which you add hot water, from the health-food store, is prepared just as quickly, but has a greater warming effect.

@ People who eat a great deal of meat need to create a balance by incorporating into their meals a lot of fresh vegetables, green leafy salads, champignons, fruit, and grain.

@ There is a method of cooking that harmonizes the entire organism. Especially when people with different constitutions and temperaments live together, it is important that the food prepared be balanced. For balanced meals, all you have to do is *combine foods and ingredients that have different thermal effects.* When you use hot spices, add refreshing fruits or vegetables. When you serve a salad as a main dish, serve a warming soup beforehand. Should you fry warming meat, sprinkle it with sprouts. Warm and refreshing foods need to be balanced. It's not a good idea to use a lot of hot spices for a while every day, even if you are a vegetarian and sensitive to coldness. Specific organs would get hot and begin to dominate other organs, which leads to an imbalance. Instead, every day use small amounts of warm spices over a longer period of time. This way, warmth energy builds up slowly and the entire organism can adjust to it. It's often best for the largest part of a meal to consist of neutral foods like whole grains and vegetables, any way you like them, because, on their own, they have a harmonizing effect on the body.

When you have been occupied for a while with the energetic, or thermal, effect of foods, you will notice one change in yourself in particular: *You will have become more intuitive in your selection of foods, asking yourself what you truly need.* Only your own body can tell you precisely what is good for you; no tables and systems can do this.

When you are cold in the winter and force yourself to have cold orange juice for breakfast, along with some toast, it's nobody's fault but your own. And the only one who will profit will be your dentist. This is because the acid from the orange juice will attack the tooth enamel if you brush your teeth half an hour before or after you have drunk the orange juice. You would probably be much happier having cooked oatmeal with stewed apples, cinnamon, and walnuts, and drinking an organic coffee with cardamom, and this actually would protect you from the cold much better!

In order to interpret the needs of the body correctly, first of all you need information. This phase calls for some brainwork. Then you need experience, that "aha!" we get when we know something from encountering it ourselves. Now the knowledge will go from the brain to your heart. Then, when you hear your inner voice and you know what to do, the knowledge has reached the belly and become second nature to you. As with my girlfriend who had so incorporated Chinese dietetics that she ate exactly what she wanted to, selecting food based on this nutritional system will become natural for you too. Even on trips and in restaurants, you will always find tasty and beneficial dishes that you can eat. And don't be shy about asking whether the meat was frozen or not. Simply say that you are allergic to frozen food and that you will faint if you eat it. You can be certain to get the truth.

The Five Elements

Wood, Fire, Earth, Metal, and Water

In order to be able to choose the right foods in each situation, you need to know about the five different tastes—sour, bitter, sweet, pungent, and salty—and the causes of illness—emotions, mental concepts, incorrect nutritional habits, weather influences, and other external factors.

The *five elements,* a Chinese system that dates back thousands of years, explains the connection between cause and effect. All mental, emotional, energetic, and material phenomena of the universe can be allocated to one of the five elements. In other words, the five elements can be viewed as an analogy system in which everything, material or abstract, finds its place according to its character and its characteristic features. This means that illness and health can be analyzed by this system as well.

We can recognize, understand, and foresee the reciprocal action and interaction of phenomena because of their cyclic nature. The five elements follow each other in a certain sequence, known as the "generative cycle." *Each life process and every human life goes through the stages of the five elements in the sequence of the generative cycle: wood, fire, earth, metal, and water.* It is up to each of us whether the potential of the respective element is fully exhausted or not.

We are born in the *wood element.* If life conditions are favorable, the foundation for creativity, spontaneity, tolerance, generosity, and openness is set in early childhood. Negative conditions can produce stiffness, intolerance, wrath, avarice, and emotional tightness, together with physical tension. All these characteristic features are allocated to the wood element.

Children who were allowed to blossom during the wood phase, who were able to develop curiosity, enthusiasm, and thirst for knowledge, have good prerequisites for fully exhausting the *fire element* in their youth. In this second phase, intelligence and knowledge, as well as intuition and mental clarity set the foundation for enjoyment of life and mental development. When the fire in us is not incited, we are disinterested, lack understanding when it comes to others, are dominated by materialism, and are incapable of unfolding a spiritual life.

Common sense, practical experience, and concentration on what is essential lead to internal and external stability, the fruit of the *earth element*, when we have reached the third phase in middle age. But when the grounding is missing, we are incapable of putting ideas

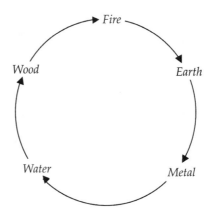

The generative cycle of the elements: Wood feeds fire, the warmth of the fire (the sun) awakens earth to life, metal is won from the earth, the minerals of the earth bring water to life, and water nourishes plants (wood).

into reality and of learning from experience. We remain noncommittal and irresponsible in relationships and feel that we do not truly belong anywhere.

In the fourth phase, associated with the *metal element*, maturity and life experience sharpen the sense for justice and the view of how things are. A material and psychological surplus, the sense of internal wealth, gives rise to the feeling of being able to give, and thus we feel less needy. This positive spiritual aspect makes us self-confident, and when there is healthy mental development as well, active compassion, the need to do something for others, develops and will continue to increase. Wise people give because they know that giving enriches them; compassionate people give because they enjoy giving. In the metal element, we are capable of recognizing the true nature of the mind amid the growing internal surplus. The mind is like space: It is empty and at the same time contains the entire potential from which everything is created. When we approach this understanding, wisdom and active compassion will develop more and more.

Existential fear as well as egotistical thinking and behavior characterize people who have not developed trust at the core of their existence. From an inability to experience the space between us as a connecting element between oneself and others comes injustice and ruthless behavior, and one will project one's own negative characteristics onto others. This space is experienced as something that divides, and a wall consisting of pride and contempt, masking our own internal weakness, manifests a shield from others.

Out of trust in the unlimited potential of the universe and of our own minds develops the understanding that the spirit cannot be destroyed. This knowledge results in fearlessness, the highest quality of the *water element*, the fifth and last stage, occurring in old age.

At this point, it is important to understand that we, on the one hand, go through the elements successively from birth to death. But, on the other hand, the potential of all the elements exists at all times in each of us and can be developed depending on external circumstances and internal abilities. The five-elements system transcends our limited sense of time; Einstein was not the first to question this.

Fear is the psychological expression of a weakened water element. It develops when we don't feel at home, don't feel safe, in the unlimited space that surrounds us. We develop defensive armor and hostility toward others in order to protect our delicate ego, losing more and more contact with our own core.

From involvement with the five elements develops wisdom and the knowledge that all phenomena in the universe are interconnected, that they depend on one another and affect one another, because matter is nothing but condensed qi, which moves and changes continuously. In part, we can understand the movements of the macrocosm from our knowledge of the microcosm. These movements follow certain laws, not unlike the cycles of the five elements. Thus, many things are foreseeable. For instance, fall is followed by winter, and as we can foresee this development, we buy warm clothing on time. Many centuries before Western calculations of time, the Chinese had already recorded certain experiences and observations, from which they recognized laws and developed from them the yin-yang model and the five-elements system.

Because we generally have not recognized our true nature, the core of our being, we must depend more or less

Allocations of the Five Elements

Element	Wood	Fire	Earth	Metal	Water
Season	Spring	Summer	Late summer	Fall	Winter
Climate	Wind	Heat	Humidity	Dryness	Cold
Color	Green	Red	Yellow	White	Black
Yin organ	Liver	Heart	Spleen	Lungs	Kidneys
Yang organ	Gallbladder	Small intestine	Stomach	Large intestine	Bladder
Sense	Seeing	Speaking	Tasting	Smelling	Hearing
Taste	Sour	Bitter	Sweet	Pungent	Salty
Emotion and attitude	Flexibility Achievement	Joy Openness	Stability Truthfulness	Sharpness Original trust	Willpower Modesty
Positive	Planning	Mental clarity	Common sense	Justice	Courage
Negative	Narrow-mindedness Irritability	Joylessness Lack of contact Wrath	Worry Sentimentality State of confusion	Sadness Inability to let go Pensiveness	Exaggerated fear Lack of motivation Being wound up

on speculation. Researchers and people who are seeking knowledge have developed their systems based on hypotheses. The theories that stand as the basis of Chinese medicine, for example, serve to help us understand the causes of illness, predict their course, and then intervene with suitable remedies.

The theory concerning the five different tastes, each of which is allocated to one of the five elements, plays a major role in Chinese dietetics. As the five pairs of internal organs are similarly allocated to the five elements, we are able to make statements about the effects of the different tastes on the organs.

On the physical level, the qi flows from organ to organ in the sequence of the *generative cycle,* in order to nourish the body and maintain organ activity. Illnesses spread in a similar manner, but in this case, the *control cycle* plays an important role. In the sections about the wood and fire elements, you'll find detailed explanations about the control cycle. In the sections about the earth, metal, and water elements, the spread of disease and the effect of different tastes within the control cycle are not discussed on their own but incorporated into the main discussion.

Wood

Wood is the first element, representing birth and childhood, as well quick growth, development, planning, and the beginning of an enterprise. It stands for the little yang of the spring, the quick upward movement of the seeds and young shoots, when the strength of the sun increases again. *The liver and gallbladder organs, the color green, the climatic factor of wind, and the sour taste are allocated to it.*

The Liver and the Gallbladder

The first-named organ of an organ pair is always the *storage, or yin, organ.* Its task is to store fluids and qi, and to supply them to the body. In the development of disease, the yin organs always play the more important role, so they are mentioned more often.

According to Chinese medicine, the liver, the first in the pair allocated to the wood element, has control over the eyes and seeing; the muscle tone, which causes the tension or slackness of the entire muscular system; the tendons; and the fingernails and toenails. It is responsible for the subtle flow of qi and its balanced distribution in the body. The liver, together with the heart and the spleen, is in large part responsible for the quantity and the quality of the blood.

Based on the control function of the respective organ, the organic cause of a disorder can be determined when symptoms occur. For example, from the point of view of TCM, eye problems when they accompany hay fever, such as itching, tears, and inflammation, are caused by a disorder of the liver's function cycle. The function cycle contains all functions of the respective organ and of the respective meridian. If you suffer from eye problems accompanying hay fever, it is a clear sign to a doctor who practices TCM that there is an energetic disorder of the liver, which must be treated for the hay fever to be cured.

Conjunctivitis also falls into this category. In this case, the doctor who practices TCM diagnoses a yang excess of the liver as the cause for the inflammation. Then the doctor goes one step further with the question of how the yang excess in the liver came about. Have anger, unpleasant stress, alcohol, pungent spices, garlic, or all of these together played a role in the process? When this question can be answered, there is the possibility of attacking the underlying cause. A means of therapy that cools the heat can support the patient effectively, taming his or her anger, so that the patient can find another way to express his or her strength potential.

Muscular tension, brittle nails, and all symptoms of blood deficiency are also consequences of a liver disorder.

Disorders in the flow of qi in the gallbladder meridian, the second area associated with the wood element, concern principally the hip, the lower back, and the pelvis area. A damp heat of the gallbladder brings about sciatica, lumbago, and hip-joint problems. Headaches on the side of the head and often migraines have the same cause. Manual meridian treatment with acupressure and acupuncture can be very helpful in such cases. People with a weak gall-bladder cannot tolerate fatty food and coffee. With them, especially the combination of sweet-fat (cream tarts, doughnuts) and salty-fat (French fries, pork) foods trigger an acute obstruction of the gallbladder.

Emotions and Mental Analogies

On the mental and emotional levels, a relaxed liver reveals itself through spontaneity, creativity, organizational skill, tolerance, and generosity. The liver hates pressure. Many neuroses develop when people are put under pressure in the wood phase, as babies or small children. They may feel pressured to achieve something, due to the excessive expectations of their parents. The liver loves relaxation and free space. Everything that grows needs space; only this way can it mature.

People with a tense liver react with irritability, anger, and rage if anyone seems to want to take away or invade their space. By expressing their anger aggressively, they try to obtain on the outside the space that is lacking on the inside. These people don't have sufficient distance to recognize that the cause for their rage lies within themselves, in their inability to create the space they need to fulfill their life tasks creatively and grow with this. But exactly herein lies the solution.

Stubbornness, obstinacy, narrow-mindedness, intolerance, and the physical tension and stiffness associated with these attitudes, can only be dissolved when we stand up for ourselves, in order to create the conditions and space where we can realize our potential and be happy. This is the ability that the wood element, with the liver and gallbladder organs, has to offer us. The liver gives us our fantasy and the contents for our life vision, as well as the courage to make plans for it and the strength to accomplish it later, in the earth element. When we try to demand the space for this from others, by complaining or putting on pressure, it is less likely that we will get it. We get the space we need rather through our wish for growth, by standing by our dreams, and by making sure that we can realize them in peace for our own good and for the good of others.

Meditative exercises like tai chi and qigong, as well as meditation, create mental calmness and internal space, because the qi, which is prone to obstructions, is activated smoothly and the person becomes more open. From this internal spaciousness, it is easier to decide whether we want to identify with the disturbing feelings of rage or preserve the feeling of calmness instead. Rage is nothing but a distortion of qi. Many Taoist and Buddhist meditation practices have the specific goal of enabling the person to transform disturbing feelings and make use of them in everyday life.

Suppressed anger, a cold rage, is difficult to deal with, as we don't experience ourselves as being angry and avoid even becoming aware of the problem. With a hot rage, the energetic base is an excess of yang, which causes the emotional outbursts. With a cold anger, the stagnation of the liver qi is in the foreground.

Those whose creativity and spontaneity are not exploited, due to a blockage of qi in the liver, are often overcome by feelings of frustration. They try to get relief through lamenting, accusing, manipulating, and controlling, and they try to create a world the way they want it to be. But these are basically useless attempts to escape from feelings of depression.

Turning to alcohol is just as unproductive. Even though alcohol, due to its pungent taste, momentarily dissolves the qi blockage and the depression, frustration hits even harder later. It is easy to understand that people with these problems feel helpless and have a hard time escaping the clutches of alcohol without therapeutic help—and even with it.

In cases of both hot and cold rage, tai chi and qigong, stretching exercises, sports without pressure, autogenic training, and meditation can be relaxing and helpful in reaching more internal distance from the intensity of the negative feelings.

Rage causes an excess of yang in the liver and/or the gallbladder. Or, conversely, it can be said that an excess of yang in these organs, due to incorrect nutrition or stress, is often accompanied by anger and rage. Regardless of which came first, it is the task of nutritional therapy to cool the heat of the liver and the gallbladder and to replenish the fluids. This will be discussed in greater detail later in connection with the different kinds of taste. But for now, here's some advice should you have an excess of yang or a qi obstruction in the liver: Stay away from garlic, all pungent-hot spices, coffee, alcohol, large quantities of meat, and rich evening meals. In addition, the qi obstruction in the liver is a problem that can be approached with acupuncture, herbal therapy, and physical exercise.

The inability to make decisions, accompanied by tension, is typically experienced by people with blockages in the gallbladder meridian. The initial cause is the qi obstruction in the liver, which spreads to the area of the gallbladder. Such blockades can be chronic, or they can occur acutely due to excessive stress or emotional conflict.

Gallbladder pain can be relieved with corn-silk tea. When drunk regularly, it has an astonishing effect on gallstones, which occur with chronic gallbladder disorders. Pour 1 quart, or liter, of hot water over 1 to 2 tablespoons of the tea, and let it steep for about 10 minutes.

Windy Weather

As the weather factor of the wood element, wind, out of all the climatic influences that trigger illness, damages the functions of the liver-gallbladder area the most. All of us have at some point experienced the effect of a draft on our bodies. Headaches, stiffness at the nape of the neck, or a stiff neck are often the consequences when we are exposed for an extended period of time to the draft of an open car or to air-conditioning. The points that run along the gallbladder meridian in the neck are appropriately called "wind gates." It is through them that wind enters the meridian and blocks the flow of qi, triggering the pains in this area. In order to prevent this, you should wear a scarf in windy weather. Wind also has the special ability of opening the surface of the body so that other damaging climatic factors can penetrate. Everyone knows that the fastest way to get a sunburn or heatstroke is when there's wind. Likewise, it is much easier to catch a head cold when the weather is not only wet and cold but also windy. If you have a distinct dislike of wind and are sensitive to drafts, you probably have a tense liver.

The Sour Taste

All foods with a sour taste are allocated to the wood element. Unripe fruit, for example, is usually green (the color of the wood element) and very sour. Ripe fruits, salad greens, vegetables, and sprouts that are green are allocated according to their taste to their respective element, but their green color is a sign that they are also characterized by the wood element. There are some foods that have a mild taste but are still, due to their direct influence on the liver and the gallbladder, assigned to the wood element. Common examples are chicken, duck, spelt, and wheat.

Here, it's important to mention that all types of meat and grain belong foremost to the sweet earth element, due to their sweet and/or mild taste and their qi-building effect. Yet some types of meat and grain have, in addition, a special effect on the organs of another element. For the sake of clarity, they are classified with the element whose organs they influence secondarily.

Almost all sour foods are refreshing, which is favorable for the wood organs, because they tend to suffer from a lack of fluids and from heat.

As discussed earlier, when there is an emotional imbalance, especially manifesting as anger and rage, the liver and the gallbladder are disturbed in their functions and heated up more than any other organs. Also, it can be said that people whose wood organs have an excess of yang or a blood deficiency, due to heating and drying foods, often react with rage, anger, and emotional fluctuations. Especially in such cases, the sour and refreshing foods are the best remedies.

The sour taste tends to make us joyful, because it cools the liver and the gallbladder. However, this is true only for the sour and refreshing foods. *Vinegar,* for instance, is sour, but not refreshing. Nevertheless, it relaxes the liver. But its quality is crucial. The value of a good, unpasteurized vinegar lies in its high content of enzymes, which activate digestion. For this reason, it is often added to certain dishes, such as lentils, at the end of the cooking process. But the vinegar must not boil; otherwise, the activity of the enzymes is destroyed. With the added vinegar, digestion is made easier; this in turn leads to a direct relaxation of the liver, which is prone to obstructions especially when digestion is overburdened.

Now we are dealing with two factors: the taste, which tells us which organ is affected primarily by the food, and the thermal effect, which tells us how the food is affecting the organ. To refresh your memory, *cold food reduces an excess of yang, refreshing food builds up blood and fluids, neutral food primarily builds up qi, warm food increases yang, and hot food combats coldness.*

Foods that are both sour and refreshing preserve and strengthen the bodily fluids and the blood. The two yin factors, blood and fluids, become damaged and reduced when yang (heat) gains the upper hand in the organs. When people take part in strenuous sports or are exposed to hot weather, causing them to sweat profusely, sour and refreshing fruit teas such as hibiscus, rose hip, and mallow ensure that the bodily fluids are not overly depleted. If a person has to work in a room that is dry and hot most of the time, such as a dry-cleaners, sour and refreshing fruits, stewed fruits, and teas balance the dryness; they do the same in cases of anger and stress.

If you have sour fruits and a wheat beer, you will calm down quickly, and the organs will become balanced again. Especially at night if you can't sleep, wheat tea can be used to calm the heart. The liver lies in front of the heart in the elements' generative cycle, and its task is to supply the heart with fluids. When there is liver heat and a deficiency of yin, this task cannot be carried out sufficiently, and internal restlessness and sleeping disorders occur.

To prepare wheat tea, cook a handful of wheat for 45 minutes in half a quart, or liter, of water. This tea harmonizes the liver and supplies the heart with fluids. The pot in which the tea is prepared should be enameled on the inside or made of clay or glass, as metal interferes with the therapeutic effect of wheat.

Basically, all whole grains have a neutral energetic, or thermal, effect, through which they harmonize the organism and build up qi. Some grains also have a slight tendency in the refreshing and warm directions, so they are classified in the respective refreshing or warm category. Barley is slightly refreshing, for example. Wheat, on the other hand, tends to be cooling. Wheat is especially suitable for building up fluids in the liver and the heart. If a person has a cold constitution, wheat should not be eaten too often.

If you want to strengthen the wood organs in particular, it makes sense to combine spelt with other wood foods such as chicken, green vegetables, and sprouts. Most vegetables have a mild taste and are allocated to the earth element. However, as the color green represents the wood element, green vegetables are a mixture of both wood and earth elements. Due to their growth, which is typical of the wood element, sprouts contain a portion of wood energy, along with earth energy. They have a refreshing effect on the liver and the gallbladder. Watercress, on the other hand, is pungent and is thus partly allocated to the metal element.

The Control Cycle

According to the theory of the five elements, one element stimulates or augments the next; this is what is known as the "generative cycle," discussed earlier. But there is also another cycle, called the "control cycle," briefly mentioned before, in which one element hinders or reduces the next. In this sequence, which is different from that of the generative cycle, wood controls earth, fire controls metal, earth controls water, and metal controls wood. The controlling element has the task of making sure that there will be no excess within the yin or yang root in the organ that it has to control. How does it do this? Either by using its yang (its warmth) to reduce an excess of yin or by using its yin (its coldness) to lessen an excess of yang. It's easy to imagine that the organ can fulfill this function if it has enough yin or yang itself. But its yin or yang may become depleted over time if it is used again and again to harmonize the next organ.

For example, it is the task of the yang of the heart to reduce the yin of the lungs when there is an excess, by means of the control cycle. A yin excess of the lungs exists when mucus is in the lungs, as when you have a head cold. Also, when a person eats too many sweets or milk products—which, due to their dampening effect, first increase the spleen's yin—an excess of the lung's yin develops. The spleen is in front of the lungs in the generative cycle and is forced to pass its excess of yin on to the lungs, because its yang is not sufficient to transform the dampness. The consequence is dampness in the lungs, with a tendency to colds with a lot of mucus. When consuming dampening foods is habitual, as is the case with "normal" children's nutrition, a decrease of the heart's yang will occur in the long run, because the heart must relinquish yang to the spleen, in order to increase its yang (the generative cycle). On the other hand, the heart uses up its yang in order to reduce the excess of yin in the lungs (the control cycle).

When a decrease in the yang of the heart occurs when there is already an excess of yin in the spleen and the lungs, digestion, mental sharpness, and concentration are weakened. In addition, there is often a craving for sweets, and one is prone to get head colds with a lot of mucus in the lungs. Try to find a kindergarten where most of the children don't suffer from this syndrome! Tropical fruits, uncooked food, cheese, yogurt, and sweeteners like sugar and honey are the cause of this. Isn't it strange that all these foods—except for sugar—are considered good for us?

The dietary therapy that is called for now is as follows: cooked grains like millet, polenta, or oats with stewed fruits and cinnamon for breakfast; meat broth with vegetables or other warming, cooked meals for lunch and dinner. After about two weeks, the craving for sweets will lessen and the chronic head colds will all but disappear. Children also become more capable of learning, have

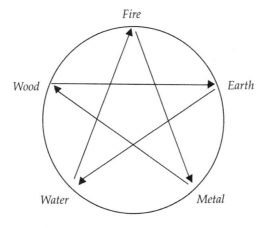

The control cycle of the elements: Wood penetrates earth, fire melts metal, earth obstructs water, metal cuts wood, water extinguishes fire.

better concentration, and are generally more vital and cheerful. Instead of watching TV, they suddenly want to go outside and play.

There is a tendency in the body for illnesses to spread from organ to organ. It is important in the therapy to stop this process, because the longer it persists the more organs are afflicted and the more difficult becomes the treatment. In such cases, balanced nutrition is the best protection. The combination of using different kinds of taste with thermal effects adapted to the seasons will balance the organism before illnesses have spread. Unfortunately, the opposite is much too common in practice, as people often exhibit heart diseases combined with kidney ailments, gallbladder problems with stomach pains, and so forth, and the connections are not being recognized.

The Effect of the Different Tastes
in the Control Cycle

The same way as the organs control each other, the taste of foods influences the yin or yang of the organs. A balanced selection of tastes keeps yin and yang in balance. Consuming an excessive amount of a certain taste will lead sooner or later to an imbalance. The sweet taste, however, is an exception, because it is naturally harmonizing. Here, "sweet" doesn't refer to intense sweetness as with chocolate, but to mild-sweet foods such as grains, vegetables, potatoes, legumes, and meat, which should constitute the largest portion of our menu.

Wood Penetrates Earth

As discussed, the wood element is associated with the sour taste. After the wood element comes the fire element, with the associated heart organ; the next one after that is the earth element, with the spleen. Concerning the influence of taste, this means that an excess of sour and cold foods increases the yin of the heart by means of the generative cycle and lowers the yang in the spleen and stomach earth organs through the control cycle. Yogurt and tropical fruits in combination, typically foods for losing weight, having sour-cold and sweet-cold properties, possess exactly this effect. The earth organs are cooled and insufficient postnatal qi is produced, so that an overall qi deficiency occurs in the long run, and a kidney-yang weakness can develop through the control cycle.

It is understood that a body weak in qi cannot produce heat to burn fat, so there is zero weight reduction. Statistics show that weight loss through consuming fewer calories is always only short-term. Logically, this diet works better for young people, because their prenatal qi is still strong enough to balance the deficiency that is caused by eating little food and generally cold food. The same is true for men, who have more yang by nature. The real problem begins for many women from age thirty-five on, and for men more likely past fifty, because now the prenatal qi is not as strong as it was when they were younger. Not only is counting calories not successful anymore, but also chronic deficiency diseases can develop. For instance, it's been seen that osteoporosis (bone decalcification) occurs most frequently in women who have kept their calorie supply down again and again over the years.

Metal Cuts Wood

There are many parallels in life to the analogy system of the five elements in the control cycle. Here are some pertaining to metal and wood: Scissors (metal) cut paper (wood), and an axe fells a tree. It's been said that we shouldn't give a knife to a friend (wood) as a gift without asking a penny for it, and we shouldn't borrow needles from a neighbor because that destroys the friendship. (Keeping up friendships is a characteristic allocated to the wood element.) According to an old superstition, we shouldn't give metal objects as a gift or lend them to friends, as they could cause an injury.

The pungent taste, associated with metal element, which controls the wood organs, is used so often that its negative effects are generally overlooked. Pungent-cold and pungent-refreshing foods like rice and radishes refresh and relax the liver, preventing an excess of yang. But too much pungent-warm and pungent-hot foods such as pungent spices, high-proof alcohol, chili, curry, garlic, and red onions lead to a yang excess of the wood organs, which is even increased further through emotional stress, time pressure, or stress on the job. With this yang excess comes a proneness to rage and anger, irritability, tension of the neck and shoulder muscles, burning of the eyes, liver inflammation, gallbladder colic, high blood pressure, and even apoplectic fits. Thus, it's clear that too much pungent-warm and pungent-hot food or alcohol can have extremely negative consequences in the long run. If you suffer from such problems, it's probably best to forgo pungent spices, strong alcohol, and especially garlic.

Garlic is not the panacea it has been chalked up to be. It is useful for arteriosclerosis, yeast infections, and cold illnesses. Yet it is quite damaging for people with liver qi stagnation, with a hot base constitution or already damaged wood organs, especially when it is eaten raw. Many people believe that they cannot cook without garlic. But don't let yourself be confined by this way of thinking. When you give up one thing, you gain another, and in this case you will be able to enjoy a whole range of flavors you had done without until now. Then when you use garlic occasionally, it is a real delight.

Fire

The fire element is associated with the great yang of the summer. Young people looking for recognition, acquiring knowledge, and researching everything have the fire character. Fire stands for mental development, inspiration, intuition, curiosity, interest, and learning. From the Chinese point of view, the earth is yin and the sky is yang. The human being stands in-between. Through our mind, we connect below and above in ourselves in a meaningful unity, as both feet are rooted firmly on the earth and we are able to reach for the stars.

The heart and small-intestine organs, the color red, the climatic factor of heat, and the bitter taste are allocated to the fire element.

The Heart and the Small Intestine

Not only do the heart and the small intestine belong to the fire element, but the Triple Burner and the cardiovascular system do as well, although they are not as important when it comes to an understanding of dietetics.

The heart controls the blood vessels and our personal radiance, which shines through the face and the eyes. It also controls our ability to present and express ourselves, as well as the tongue and speaking. The heart is called the "emperor of the organs." All disturbances and positive influences that take place in another organ are registered by the heart and made visible by means of the tongue. This is the reason why tongue diagnosis plays such a major role in TCM. For the early recognition of heart disease, it is especially important.

The radiance of the face and the eyes mirrors the condition of the heart. You have probably been asked if you were in love when you looked especially good. Or vice versa: When you were in love, you most likely got compliments on your glowing appearance. The ability to express oneself verbally, to fascinate others and to keep their interest, lies in the strength of the heart. In order to enforce what we have said, or to declare our love and sincerity, we put our hand onto our heart.

When the heart yang is weakened, we speak very slowly or do not want to communicate at all. If there is heart heat or a deficiency of fluids, we talk a lot and very fast and sometimes in a confused manner. Disorders of heart energy have an influence on sleep. Difficulties in falling asleep and in being able to sleep through the night are a sign of a deficiency of blood, yin, or heat of the heart.

The small intestine, as the partner organ of the heart, has a subordinate position when illnesses develop due to errors in nutrition. This is because these illnesses are strongly connected to the pathology of the entire digestive tract and are treated together with the disorders of the spleen in dietetic practice.

The small intestine, however, has a special function, which can be the explanation for recurrent *bladder problems* not caused by bacteria. Time pressure is a stress factor that produces heat in the heart. In order to protect the heart, it is one of the tasks of the small intestine to divert this heat by way of the bladder. This process causes burning and pain when a person urinates, and can be a cause for a bladder infection. From the perspective of therapeutic nutrition, it is a matter of cooling the heart through refreshing food. You also need to stop drinking coffee. In the long run, it will be necessary to reduce the heavy demands and the time pressure.

Emotions and Mental Analogies

The heart is the seat of the spirit. Love, compassion, and wisdom are its characteristic features, which emerge more and more through development, affecting our actions and behavior. When we realize that all people basically want the same thing, which is to be happy and avoid suffering, and that people behave well when they are doing well, and bad when they are doing bad, we are not far from developing an empathy and an active compassion for others. Openness, a readiness for communication, and a real interest in others create a sense of delight and the feeling of inner wealth, which we want to share with others. When we lend our life a deep, useful meaning this way, our heart is strengthened automatically.

Enjoyment and laughter belong to the fire element. The highest form of enjoyment is created independently of external conditions, so it can't be unsettled by rainy weather or by other unfavorable circumstances. The ability to preserve a cheerfulness of the heart and an internal smile in all circumstances of life is the result of many Taoist and Buddhist spiritual practices.

Try this simple exercise: Focus more on the characteristics of a person that you like and less on the traits that you dislike. This way, you will discover many positive things that you just weren't aware of before. Possibly now and then you will have to deal with a person in whom you cannot see anything positive at all. Don't be deterred by this; you will find something. For example, if the person is wearing a nice tie, and you can bear to give him a compliment on it, the tables can turn. You suddenly see friendly traits where you had only met with defenses. The Buddhist practice of cultivating a pure heart in everyday life is so simple and effective, because all people, in fact, carry love and wisdom in themselves, when you help them to discover this.

Yet anyone who looks critically for mistakes will find weaknesses and errors everywhere. By reversing the polarity of our focus, however, we will gradually come to see that things do not exist separately from the observer, that the way we look at the world determines in large part what we perceive. A difficult situation can always also be experienced as a challenge, which makes us strong and offers possibilities for growth. And beautiful, touching experiences show us the potential of the human spirit.

Although both Taoism and Buddhism are practiced in China, the medical philosophy and the health consciousness of the Chinese are mainly rooted in Taoist ideas, as they were already thousands of years old when Buddhism first appeared in China. A basic component of Taoist spiritual practice is the goal of strengthening health, prolonging life, and increasing overall well-being. The effects of the Taoist health exercises that were handed down and still thrive today, to which tai chi and qigong belong, are unique and quietly powerful, when taught and conveyed in the correct manner.

In contrast to the Taoist orientation with its focus on the health of the body, the Buddhist way is directed toward the mind, here and now, as well as concerned with karma beyond death. The fruit of Buddhist practice depends a great deal on its uninterrupted transmission through a line of enlightened teachers, making the teacher-student relationship very important. Even in China today, Taoist adepts are quick to acknowledge that Buddhism's achievements regarding direct work with the mind are outstanding.

Spiritual recognition, but also thirst for knowledge, openness to new things, and pleasure in learning are the best guarantees for a long and healthy life, as well as for a healthy heart. There are many elderly people whose mental faculties and openness to new things have not diminished and who enjoy an active and meaningful old age.

The heart requires one more thing: that we take our time; that we take time in order to have time; that we take leisure time; that we take time to reflect, to think about whether or not we really want to be doing what we are doing. Take time to look inward, to enjoy, to see the small things, because the small things are just as important as the large ones, and the hidden things just as significant as the obvious.

Time is associated with the fire element. The heart suffers most from time pressure. Aside from mental and emotional exhaustion, stress most frequently leads to heart heat or lack of fluids. In addition, an already existing deficiency of liver blood in combination with stress can develop into a blood deficiency of the heart in the long run. The consequences of this are nervousness, fear, sleeping disorders, bladder infections, heart disease, and ulcers in the small intestine. Conversely, it can be said that lack of sleep weakens the fluids of the heart.

The feeling of not being understood usually goes hand in hand with the inability to make oneself understood. This and other difficulties in expressing oneself, such as stuttering, are disorders in the area of the heart and small intestine, as are conditions of confusion and mental illnesses.

Hot Weather

Heat is the climatic factor that attacks the heart most severely. When the sun shines intensely, it is important to protect the head, because the sun penetrates here most quickly into the body. Do what you can to prevent sunburn; possible damage to the skin and the danger of skin cancer should be reason enough. However, the heat not only affects the surface of the skin, but it also penetrates deep into the body and can cause disturbances there, which often only after months produce symptoms and disorders. Suddenly, a high fever, a flu-like condition, or skin diseases can develop. If then merely the symptoms are treated and the heat is not directed out of the body, chronic diseases can occur.

The Bitter Taste

Foods with a bitter taste belong to the fire element, as do other foods like buckwheat, rye, lamb, and goat. The taste of red foods such as sweet cherries, red grapes, and red pepper is associated with the earth element, but due to their red color these foods also have an energetic influence on the organs of the fire element.

The bitter taste directs the qi downward. Bitter herbs, contained in teas for the gallbladder, for example, have a cooling effect, and they also assist in the transport of the contents of the stomach and the intestine, which is directed downward. Especially a gallbladder with a tendency toward heat and stagnation is relaxed through the downward movement, and its flow is stimulated as well. This effect is also favorable for the digestion of fat, which is made more difficult when there is a disorder of the gallbladder. This downward movement is an important support when it comes to all digestive problems.

Aperitifs often have a bitter taste in order to stimulate digestion, just as a lot of kitchen herbs do. Bitter liqueurs are drunk after the evening meal in order to mobilize the process of digestion, especially after eating rich food.

Bitter and cold salads consisting of radicchio, endive, and chicory, for example, and cold-refreshing fire and wood foods and beverages, like grape juice with hot water, help to cool the heat in the heart and to build up fluids. This is particularly so in cases of exhausting mental exertion and stress. Bitter and warm beverages, such as coffee, hot chocolate, and red wine, and herbs, like rosemary, thyme, and oregano, are drying. In humid weather, however, they protect the body from dampness. In the generative cycle, the earth element, with the spleen and stomach organs, follows the fire element. The spleen suffers most from dampness. In the right quantity, the bitter-warm taste strengthens the qi of the spleen and prevents an accumulation of dampness.

Yet consuming an excessive amount of bitter-warm foods and beverages like coffee and red wine can lead to a lack of fluids and to heat of the heart. This in turn can give rise to the same conditions through which stomach ulcers can develop. Generally, the bitter-warm taste and roasted stimulants like coffee and hot chocolate should be avoided in all cases of substance-deficiency disorders, like sleeping problems, loss of hair, and osteoporosis (bone decalcification). They should also be avoided when there are blood-deficiency and circulation ailments, as they deplete the blood even more and harden the blood vessels.

Coffee is a drug that is healing in small quantities and harmful in large quantities. In most people, a strong need for coffee has to do with a qi deficiency of the spleen and a yang deficiency of the kidneys. Coffee warms these organs, with short-term effects on fatigue, lack of concentration, and internal coldness. But the deficiencies of qi and yang, which are the underlying causes of these problems, are certainly not eliminated; drinking coffee merely temporarily obscures the symptoms concealing the actual problems.

The Control Cycle

Fire controls metal, and the lungs and the large intestine are the organs allocated to the metal element. Through the control cycle, an excess of stimulants such as coffee and cigarettes causes a yin deficiency of the lungs and the large intestine. The lungs are responsible for the functions of the skin. A yin deficiency of the lungs dries out the skin, aging it prematurely. If you want to retain the smoothness and the youthful appearance of your skin, as well as the health of your lungs, try to stay away from coffee and cigarettes. Many people say that coffee stimulates digestion. The reason for this is the draining effect of the bitter taste. However, in the long run, drinking a lot of coffee dries out the large intestine and constipation can result.

Black tea and green tea are both drying, especially when it comes to the yin of the heart. The fact that these teas are stimulating is due to this effect, as the yang of the heart automatically steps forward when the yin is reduced, which makes us feel stimulated mentally.

Green tea is cooler than black tea. The Chinese people drink green tea almost continuously, and it agrees with them. This is because they eat cooked food most of the time, selecting the food for each meal according to their constitution and the season; thus, the cooling effect of the tea, which especially acts upon the kidney yang, is balanced. But if you are frequently cold anyway, it's best to stay away from green tea. The way we drink green tea usually consists of making fresh cups, but in China they do it differently. They put a little less than a teaspoon of tea into the cup and pour hot water over the same tea for hours. As the tea becomes thinner and thinner, the bodily fluids, which were dried out by the first strong infusion, are restored.

Green tea is an old and trusted remedy for damp heat, meaning dampness that stagnates inside and causes heat. People who are prone to water retention and have heat symptoms at the same time (an excess of yang) find green tea an excellent means to divert dampness out of the body. Being overweight, accompanied by a strong hunger and a dark-yellow coloration of the urine, is an indication of damp heat.

The drying effect of black tea can be beneficial for the spleen when used reasonably—one to two cups a day—in cases of dampness. On the other hand, it is advised to avoid black tea if your eyes are swimming, your eyes are sensitive to light, or you are prone to muscle cramps, because it increases the already existing blood deficiency even more.

Earth

Earth is the nourishing, balancing element that glides throughout the year, harmoniously forming a transition between the seasons. The humidity in nature is associated with the earth element. Humidity and our own bodily fluids are the origin of the nourishing yin that helps create substance and thus life with the help of qi. Among the seasons, late summer—the time of harvest—is allocated to the earth element.

Earth is the element of middle age. Maturity, stability, and the wish to actualize our goals lead to establishing a foundation for a career and a family. A child needs a secure, safe place to be able to develop and thrive. The basic instincts of mothers and of women in general are to create and preserve a home. Possibly this is why women usually handle money more carefully and strive more for security than men.

The spleen and stomach organs, the color yellow, the climatic factor of humidity or rain, and the sweet taste are allocated to the earth element.

The Spleen

In traditional Chinese medicine, when we talk about the spleen, we actually mean the spleen and the pancreas, as well as their common meridian. In ancient China, it was prohibited to cut open corpses, so the anatomical facts on which Western medicine is based were not known in Chinese medicine. The overall function of the spleen and the pancreas and their meridian makes up what Chinese medicine calls today the "function cycle of the spleen/pancreas."

The spleen and stomach earth organs have, as mentioned earlier, the important task of extracting qi from food in order to produce the body's own postnatal qi. The spleen is the "empress over the fluids." It is responsible for nourishing and adding moistness to the tissue and muscles, and for distributing the bodily fluids. Its control function over muscles and tissue can be deduced from this. Whereas the liver controls muscle tone, the spleen nourishes muscles, thus determining their strength.

When people get bruises easily or if they have cellulite, this is likely because of a qi weakness of the spleen. Furthermore, fatigue and a lack of concentration occur, because a weak spleen does not produce enough nutrition qi and the entire organism is weakened. A craving for sweets develops, for the sweet taste nourishes the spleen, and the spleen has control over the sense of taste. This way, the body is able to announce what it is lacking and to demand the right taste. Whether we interpret this need correctly and satisfy it, is another question.

Other signs are cold hands and a pale complexion, because the lack of qi slows down the blood flow, so the periphery is not nourished sufficiently anymore. When the spleen's yang is weak and water is retained, subcutaneous fatty layers develop on the buttocks, hips, and upper thighs. Also, the person is generally overweight, because the metabolism has slowed down. Soft stools, partially with undigested food remains, is a sign that food is not being utilized and the body is not being supplied sufficiently with nutrients and qi. The digestive tract is weak and cold; therefore, a lack of appetite, flatulence and bloating, and the feeling of being overly full occur. During the day, the person often breaks out in a sweat without having done anything strenuous. This has to do with the spreading of the qi deficiency and the weakening of the Upper Burner, or the lungs. Also, now that the qi is neglecting its control over the skin, there is no strength to keep the pores closed.

As the cooling process continues, a yang deficiency (a state of coldness) develops from the spleen's lack of qi. The stool becomes watery, the frequency of defecation increases, and one's overall exhaustion worsens, because meanwhile the other organs have become affected by the lack of qi as well. Abdominal pains can develop, as can prolapses, such as a prolapse of the uterus, due to the weakness of the connective tissue.

The result of a chronic lack of qi in the spleen is frequently a blood deficiency, with such symptoms as night blindness, sensitivity to light, limbs that have fallen asleep, emotional vulnerability, and sleep disorders. This is because postnatal qi is the basis for blood production. In the further course of a yang weakness of the Lower Burner, a yang deficiency of the kidneys develops in many cases when a person consumes a lot of uncooked food, cold fruits, refined white sugar, and ice-cold beverages. Now not only are the hands cold, but the feet, knees, hips, and buttocks as well. After lying down all night, there's frequently back pain early in the morning, which improves with movement. Also, the person has to urinate more at night, and there is a decrease in libido. Overall, it can be said that the condition is one of exhaustion and joylessness.

Unbalanced Nutrition and Incorrect Eating Habits

There are many causes of a lack of qi. Foremost is consuming qi-less, cooling, overly moistening, and difficult-to-digest foods, but eating habits geared toward gratifying short-term desires, unbalanced nutrition, and weight-loss diets also play a role. And, ironically, quite often following the well-meaning advice of therapists and counselors based on the latest findings in the study of nutrition can have the same result.

Many people nowadays seriously try to eat healthily. It is because of confusing, half-true, and often exaggerated information, however, that people who are conscious of good nutrition often go in the completely opposite direction. And today's nutrition systems fail to take into account the energetic effect of food, the thermal effect, and the food's digestibility. Because people tend to believe blindly in science, and people who need help often try to act in good faith, they continue to eat a certain diet, even when they realize that this way of eating is not good for them. In addition, the initiator of the new health diet might have said from the beginning that the change in diet might well be accompanied by feelings of indisposition. In such cases, it is hard to tell just how long these feelings will last and whether or not they have anything to do with the new food not being wholesome and thus weakening the organism.

The main problem of most modern diets is that the energy aspect, the thermal effect of food, is neglected completely. All methods based on Western nutrition recommend too much raw food, too many milk products, and too many tropical fruits, which lead to yang weakness and an increase in dampness. The Middle Burner, the spleen, is weakened as a result, and this in turn is detrimental to the production of postnatal qi.

Ill Due to a "Healthy" Diet

Many of the following foods and eating habits are recommended in various diet trends. But when the foods are consumed regularly and the eating habits taken to the extreme, a qi deficiency of the spleen can result. So, be leery of the following:

- Cheese, milk, yogurt, and other sour-milk products
- Raw or uncooked food
- Large amounts of fruit, especially tropical fruit like bananas, oranges, and kiwis; fruit juices
- Ice-cold beverages and water
- Large quantities of any beverage, drunk even though you are not thirsty

@ Fasting; no breakfast

@ For breakfast, having melted-cheese sandwiches or jam on toast, cold cereal with milk, or just raw fruit

The recommendation to eat only raw fruit in the morning is ridiculous advice for a number of reasons. First of all, there are just a small percentage of people with whom this agrees. In addition, most people who eat only fruit for breakfast, an idea propagated in a recent book that sold millions of copies, damage their spleen qi and kidney yang. This in turn decreases their vitality, ability to achieve, joy in living, sexual desire, and overall quality of life, especially as they age. The weakness in the spleen and the kidneys promotes allergies in children whose mothers followed this diet before or during pregnancy, or weakened their spleen in some other way. In addition, mycosis of the intestine is promoted and the immune system is weakened.

This recommendation is based on the premise that digestion is particularly weak in the morning and that fruit is the most digestible food. The opposite is closer to the truth, however, as fruit is not especially digestible and digestion is probably the strongest in the morning. According to the Chinese "organ clock," which describes the cyclical changes of the individual organs' qi over the course of twenty-four hours, the qi reaches its highest point between seven and eleven in the morning in the function cycles of the spleen and the stomach, meaning in the digestive tract. Thus, the morning is the best time to absorb all the qi needed for an active day from the food we eat. For this reason, a wholesome, warm breakfast consisting of spicy or sweet cooked grain or soup is best.

Ill Due to Dietary Mistakes and Processed Food

When people are unaware of proper nutrition or acceptable quantities, certain foods and eating habits can lead to a qi deficiency of the spleen. Therefore, be cautious when it comes to the following:

- Refined sugar and all food products containing it: Sweets, chocolate, baked goods, ketchup (contains up to 45 percent sugar), lemonade, soft drinks, instant hot chocolate
- Foods containing phosphates: Lemonade, soft drinks, juices, melted-cheese dishes, sausage, smoked goods
- Qi-less, overly processed food: Canned food, pre-prepared meals, packaged products like sauces, soups, and spice mixtures, baking mixes, bread, rolls, light products, highly refined flour, noodles, frozen food from the supermarket
- Food that you froze yourself and frozen food from the health-food store: Meat, vegetables, bread, butter, etc.
- Food and beverages prepared or heated up in the microwave
- Butter from the supermarket (most of the milk is frozen and heated up in the microwave)
- Ice-cold beverages
- Cheese sandwiches
- Forgoing cooked meals in general

Dampness Suffocates the Qi of the Spleen (Yin Excess)

A deficiency of qi in the spleen always goes hand in hand with an inadequate distribution of the bodily fluids and with the development of dampness, especially from eating too many milk products (except for butter) and sweets. Butter from the health-food store builds up qi, does not cause mucus, and thus is a high-quality food product, in contrast to margarine. But milk products, chocolate, even honey, and all other sweeteners add dampness to the body.

There are differences in consistency when it comes to dampness. Over time, dampness can thicken and becomes mucus. Chocolate in particular produces a toxic, hot, tough form of mucus, as the cocoa portion is warm in its thermal effect and the moisture from the milk and sugar parts transforms into thick mucus. The result is an obstruction in the qi flow. Milk products give rise to a dampness that "suffocates" the spleen. The qi flow is also blocked through this, and water is retained in the organs and tissue.

This can be a cause for being overweight, chronic inflammation of the mucous membranes, cold illnesses especially in small children, bronchitis, sinus infections, and allergic reactions. The fluid in the tissue leads to cellulite on the upper thighs and the buttocks, to water retention in the face especially in the morning, and to swollen hands.

The excess of yin in the spleen, described here, goes hand in hand with the following symptoms as well: a heavy feeling in the arms and legs, mental numbness, depression, lack of thirst, bloating, soft stools, and sometimes nausea. When the dampness reduces the kidney fire, exhaustion and water retention in the legs up to the hip occur, as well as all other signs of a deficiency of yang. Dampness that is combined with heat can affect the gall-bladder and lead to colic and gallstones. Generally, it can be said that any food that is hard to digest produces mucus in the long run.

The Stomach: Our Strongest Organ

The stomach tolerates a great deal, and it takes a long time until signs of illness show up. Together with the large intestine, it forms an internal protective shield against illness. The external protection is the resistance energy, the wei qi, controlled by the lungs, which enfolds the body like an invisible cover. Once this protection fails, however, a superficial ailment like a head cold can develop. If the cold is not treated or is treated incorrectly—for example, by suppressing the fever—then there is a possibility that it will penetrate inside. There, the original banal ailment can develop into a chronic illness. The internal resistance of the stomach and the large intestine tries to prevent this from happening.

The Chinese have this saying: "As long as the earth organs are healthy, every illness can be healed." This is because the stomach, together with the spleen, is the source of postnatal qi. Situated at the center, the earth organs are the postnatal base of life and are responsible for resistance.

Cooling food and cold beverages, especially with ice cubes, weaken the stomach's qi. The same holds true for irregular and hasty meals, serious conversations during meals (think of business lunches), ice-cold beverages with meals, food that is too hot, and stress. A young, robust person will be able to withstand all of these factors at first, but *the small bad habits are what produce the big problems in the long run.*

A qi weakness of the stomach generally will not be noticed for a long time, as only minimal restrictions crop up at the beginning. For example, you may only be able to eat small quantities at a time; when eating larger quantities, you may feel overly full or slightly nauseous. Sometimes there is an aversion to cold beverages and food. If the qi weakness develops into stomach coldness, you may have such symptoms as stomach pains, belching or vomiting of clear stomach fluid, and a strong aversion to cold beverages.

Heating foods and beverages, such as pungent spices, very browned meat, coffee, red wine, and high-proof alcohol, are causes of stomach heat. There are also certain eating habits that bring on stomach heat, like eating before going to sleep, eating too much meat in the evening, consuming overly large portions at meals, and continuous snacking. Other culprits are emotional stress or stress on the job and overexertion. These factors block the liver qi, and thus the descent of the stomach qi, which leads to food stagnation, rotten food in the stomach, and too much acidity. Bad breath, especially in the morning, is a clear sign of this.

Stomach heat can be detected from having a strong appetite along with bouts of ravenous hunger, so it is one of the causes for being overweight. But it all depends on one's constitution, as there are people with stomach heat who can eat everything in sight and not put on any weight at all. Other signs of stomach heat are painful bleeding of the gums, sour belching, burning stomach pain, constipation, and strong thirst with a preference for cold beverages.

A lack of stomach fluids is the result of a heat illness or an overall deficiency of yin. The symptoms of this are a dry mouth especially just after waking up, a loss of appetite despite having been hungry, a problem digesting food, belching, and constipation.

Nutrition Style

How we select and prepare food shows up most notably in the strength or the weakness of the earth organs. But another factor also plays an important role, which can be called our "nutrition style." If every morning you are disgruntled and tense as you stare into yet another bowl of cooked whole-grain cereal, yearning for pancakes with sausages, you are not obeying one of the highest commands of good nutrition style, which is *to enjoy our meals.* Take time for your breakfast, and try to find something that is not only healthy but also appeals to you.

In addition, try to avoid serious discussions or arguments during meals. This means no or at least less "business dinners." It's been found that people who regularly work mentally during dinner or whose emotions are tense become ill. From about seventh grade on, most of us have seen that eating before a test is detrimental to our intellectual powers, as the blood goes to the stomach, where it is needed for digestion. If we force ourselves mentally while eating, problems with digestion are bound to follow.

It's also important *to eat as soon as you get hungry.* When you delay eating for a long time, the spleen qi is weakened, and you will eat more than is good for you later on. We are creatures of habit. Just as you may have gotten used to not eating the entire day, you can get accustomed to eating regularly again.

Pay attention at your favorite restaurant to how you feel after your meal. The taste is not the only important factor; the food must also agree with you. If you do not feel pleasantly nourished, but simply full, after the meal, find another restaurant. Also, enjoy a gourmet meal once in a while, not just all the time.

If you feel that you may have become overly obsessed

with food, and that everything in your life now seems to revolve around that, then ask yourself: Do I want to eat in order to live, or live in order to stick to nutrition rules? And finally I want to warn you of a mistake people often make when they have gotten involved in a new program. For example, because you now know how harmful refined sugar is, don't spoil it for your best friend or colleague when they order chocolate mousse for dessert. The best rule of thumb is to give advice only when asked. And that is bound to happen when you make a joyful and healthy impression as a result of your new eating habits.

Emotions and Mental Analogies

Earthbound people are distinguished foremost through their stability, healthy common sense, and practical nature. They take charge of their life, can be relied upon, and help out when it is necessary. They do not have any interest in building castles in the air or in having high-blown philosophical discussions. On the other hand, they are always a good sport and know the right direction to go in. They are ideal business partners, because what they do is to the point and constant.

When the earth element is too heavy, however, people tend to be narrow-minded, stubborn, intolerant, and inflexible. They believe only what they see and do not take any risks. Their possessions are their security, and their primary interest in life is to increase them.

On the other hand, people with a deficiency of the earth element are generally creative but rather reckless; they tend to be dreamers, yet unfortunately their dreams often get botched in their execution. One can philosophize with them night after night and have a lot of fun. However, as business partners, they are completely unsuitable, as they have too much fire. Yet when earth and fire offset each other to a certain extent, people are generally well balanced. They function well in everyday life and use their brain.

When the spleen's qi is weak, we have a tendency to ponder, to think in circles, to worry, and to imagine all kinds of things that can happen. This unnecessary mental effort usually resolves around us. Women in middle age tend to have this problem, for their spleen is just beginning its decline, and they may not have any important life work anymore because their children are grown and have left home. Through constant pondering, the spleen is weakened, and a tendency toward depression can develop.

From the Chinese point of view, women around the age of fifty experience a sense of new energy that they can use in the outside world, in order to become active in a way that is meaningful for them and that gives them pleasure. Many women this age start a new project or quit their profession so that they can pursue something that gives them more satisfaction.

The ability to focus, whether in the sense of mental work or perceiving what is essential, relies on the strength of the spleen. People who work at keeping their powers of concentration with increasing age also improve their inner stability and evenness of temper. Absentmindedness is a condition of our times. We are constantly occupied with our thoughts and ignore what is right in front of our nose. Holistic health and meditation exercises help us regain our inner stability and calmness, and thus the ability to clearly perceive what is happening at the moment. A Chinese Buddhist monk, after having meditated for twenty years, said something to this effect: "Now the spirit is finally there where the behind is sitting."

Humid or Rainy Weather

Everyone knows how depressing it can be in the fall when it rains for three weeks in a row. It is typical for dampness to sink down and pull our moods down with it. It can lead to paralyzing fatigue and depression not only in rainy-and-cold climatic zones but also in humid-and-warm tropical regions.

Some years ago, I participated in a course at a very beautiful seminary house in the Allgäu region of Bavaria. The house and the neighboring village had one big disadvantage, though. They were located directly at the foot of the northern side of a mountain. The most fantastic healing herbs were growing on the slope, but there was never any sun. The entire area was misty. After some of us experienced nausea and diarrhea, we found out that a number of people in this area had been suffering from these problems for many years and didn't know what to do about it.

When people are exposed to moisture for a long time due to the climate or a damp apartment or workplace, protecting themselves from it becomes difficult. But even when we are exposed to dampness for a brief period of time, it can penetrate the body and thus make us ill, especially when we are susceptible to it, due to a spleen qi weakness.

The spleen of many women is weakened before and during menstruation. So, it's especially important for women to protect themselves during that time of the month. Wet hair, a wet bathing suit, or clammy clothing from working out at the gym can cause an acute dampness disorder such as diarrhea; then the dampness can penetrate into the body deeper, thus leading to susceptibility. People who suffer from an excess of yin have, as a natural protective reaction, a strong aversion to rain and muggy weather.

The Sweet Taste

Many earth foods have a yellowish or brownish color: Pumpkin, carrots, sweet potatoes, and raw sugar, for example, fall into this category. Yellowish and brownish legumes have a strong share of the earth element, but because of their energetic effect on the kidney and bladder water organs they are allocated to the water element.

The mild-sweet taste, as it occurs in grains, potatoes, meat, and so forth, nourishes, harmonizes, and moistens the organism. It strengthens the body by building up qi and moistens it by stimulating the production of fluids. Through the supply of fluids and the slowdown of the energetic process, which is also caused by sweet foods, people are better able to relax and handle stress. In line with the position of the earth element, sweetness is the taste at the center. Unlike foods with other predominant tastes, foods that are mildly sweet can almost be lived on exclusively without causing any imbalance. In fact, sweet foods ensure that the organs are supplied evenly and are balanced.

Wonderful! We can all live on cakes and cookies! From now on, you never have to cook anymore! Unfortunately, this is not the case. Everything said until now about the sweet taste refers essentially to the large group of grains, to legumes, to vegetables containing starch, and to those types of meat that are kept in their natural state but are cooked. On the other hand, foods that have been overly processed, like sweets made with white flour and refined sugar, have thus lost their ability to provide healthy nourishment.

Sugar is a qi thief. Most of the leading experts on nutrition may not know anything about qi, but they all seem to be in agreement for once about the harmful effects of sugar. But why then do we crave sweets especially when we are unable to concentrate or when we are over-strained or tired? The answer is very simple: After all, the body does not say, "I want chocolate." It merely says that it wants something sweet. Millet, eggs, potatoes, and beef broth are all sweet foods that build up qi. The stronger the need for sweet things, the weaker is the qi and the spleen, or the greater is the inner tension. When women eat sweets often, the cause is mostly a qi deficiency of the spleen; for men, it is rather inner tension.

The spleen and the stomach make their shortage known directly through the development of the need for something sweet. The liver does something similar, but less frequently, by asking for sour foods, when it is tense or there is a lack of fluids, as during pregnancy. When it comes to the kidneys, it sometimes asks to be hardened with the help of something salty should there be a yang deficiency (the kidneys love hardness, which is achieved with the drying effect of salt).

When your body is telling you that it needs something sweet, it is up to you to make the correct interpretation. There are many healthy sweet foods that will satisfy the cravings in acute cases if you are determined to forgo for the most part sweets containing refined sugar. It is important, as a wise precaution, to store some healthy sweet foods in your cupboards so that you don't run to the bakery or even to a convenience store at night. Dried fruit and nuts, health bars, and snacks sweetened with honey from the health-food store should always be on hand during the first phase of giving up sugar. Your nutrition must be changed gradually to neutral, warm, and cooked food, and then the ravenous craving for sweet things will disappear. But this usually takes a few days. When the body has built up enough qi and is being supplied with healthy sweet food, a slice of cake or a piece of chocolate is allowed again. But until then, you need to be disciplined. Even if you eat foods with the highest nutritional content, the body isn't able to build up enough qi when you consume sugar every day.

From the viewpoint of nutritional science, valuable nutrients, minerals, and vitamins are extracted from the body through the transformation of white cane sugar. In addition, intense variations of the blood-sugar level can occur, which can lead to the outbreak of diabetes when we get older, should we have a predisposition for it. Sugar not only creates an ideal environment for damaging bacteria to develop around the teeth, but also in the intestine, which causes an imbalance in the intestinal flora. This is the basis for the development of intestinal fungal infections, skin diseases, and other toxic processes.

From the perspective of Chinese medicine, sugar destroys the qi of the spleen and the yang of the kidneys, thus damaging the area of the spleen and the pancreas through constant overstrain. In addition, sugar has a cooling effect, which causes a cooling of the earth organs.

Sugar is addictive. This is how the process works: Because our energy level increases only for a short time—about twenty minutes—when we eat sweets, and then sinks below the previous energy level, this causes in us a need for even more sugar. An addiction is always a compulsion and a constraint. For a lot of people, having to live without sugar seems like an impossible restriction. In reality, it is more a matter of ending a constricting, compulsive habit, in order to be able to choose freely and spontaneously from the wide variety of foods available; this is real freedom!

Grains and honey are both foods of high quality. But when a food is very sweet, as are honey, maple syrup, and raw sugar, for example, there is easily the danger of the spleen becoming too damp and of its digestion function becoming damaged. If you want to eat healthily, sooner or later you'll need to include whole grains in your diet. Whole grains like brown rice or millet are easy to prepare and extremely versatile to use. They can be stored raw or cooked and can be combined with many other foods. Whether sweet or salty, ground or used whole, they can form the basis for incredibly diversified meals.

Millet and corn, in the form of corn semolina (polenta), which is available throughout the year, as well as toasted oat flakes are very good for strengthening the earth organs. Breakfast is the ideal meal for putting your good resolutions into practice. Cook enough millet or polenta to last for two or three days. In the morning, just stew some local fruits briefly in fruit juice. Now add the prepared grain or oat flakes. Dried fruit, raisins, nuts, and cinnamon can be sprinkled on top to complete the meal. Millet mixed with a boiled egg and some butter, nutmeg, and salt also makes for a hearty morning meal. If you are not very hungry in the morning, take some of your cooked muesli (cereal consisting of oats, nuts, and fruit) with you to work. It also tastes great cold, and it satisfies any craving for sweet things and does not put on fat. Grain has the advantage of being transformed very slowly in the body (two to four hours), so normally no feeling of hunger develops before then. Therefore, grains are the ideal food for losing weight.

I have witnessed over and over again people, but especially women, who have gone hungry for years on diets achieve success finally when they change their diet to cooked grain meals with vegetables, meat, and a little fat. These successes occur when the cause of the weight problem is a qi deficiency of the spleen. The wholesome food supplies the body with enough qi to burn fat and to avoid the hunger between meals as well as the craving for sweets. The result is a harmonizing of the entire organism, in addition to losing weight.

In order to benefit from these recommendations, however, you need to be aware that there are two types of people with differently functioning metabolisms. The first type eats grains in combination with something sweet like fruit and doesn't become hungry again for hours. The second type becomes famished after one or two hours having eaten the same sweet dish. If you are the second type, you will do better if you eat a small amount of meat, legumes, or fat—instead of something sweeter—together with a small amount of grains or with vegetables, as the protein or the fat is more sustaining.

Wheat has a cooling effect, and *spelt* (a hard-grained form of wheat) a neutral to slightly warming influence. Both grains build up qi and harmonize the liver, the gallbladder, and the heart. Brown rice has the same effect on the lungs, the large intestine, the kidneys, the liver, and the gallbladder. It is especially suitable for relaxing the wood organs, by reducing superfluous heat and replenishing fluids. Oats have a stimulating and warming effect on the spleen, the stomach, the lungs, and the large intestine. And rye harmonizes the heart and the spleen.

In addition, all cooked whole grains rid the entire organism of toxins. In other words, anyone who eats whole grains can permit him- or herself a few unhealthy detours without experiencing damage right away. The excretion of toxic deposits brought about by eating whole grains is especially important for people who frequently eat meat, drink coffee, and consume sweets. However, because the environment is so badly polluted, everyone benefits from this repetitive cleansing of toxins.

Sweet-cold and sweet-refreshing vegetables, fruits, and fruit juices protect the heart and the stomach from heat by moistening and cooling the earth organs. This effect, in the correct amount, is especially helpful in the summer if your intellect is strained or you have trouble sleeping. In addition, these foods moisten the large intestine, which helps in cases of constipation. They replenish the fluids of the lungs, and therefore are helpful for a dry cough that often develops from heavy cigarette smoking or drinking a lot of coffee. Through the control cycle, they prevent excessive kidney fire, which expresses itself through hyperactivity and excessive sexual desire.

Yet the correct amount is crucial. Too much sweet-cold food depletes the qi in the spleen and the stomach, cools the yang in the heart, and thus hinders mental activity, especially the ability to express oneself. In addition, the lungs become overly damp, so head colds can develop; the digestive tract is stretched, which causes sluggishness in the intestine; and the kidneys cool off by means of the control cycle, leading to inner coldness and fatigue as well as reducing sexual desire.

Meat generally has a strong earth quota. But various types of meat also affect the organs of other elements, so they are categorized with these respective elements. Meat, on principle, builds up qi. Beef belongs to the earth element and is neutral. When it is browned strongly and when spices are used, it has an additionally warming effect. Therefore, beef is ideal for building up the qi of the spleen. Small quantities of meat, homemade broths, and

soups are best. The broth can then be used in the preparation of other meals. This way, you can build up qi without
eating meat every day.

Sweet-warm foods such as carrots, pumpkin, and fennel
warm and strengthen the spleen, the lungs, the large intestine, and the kidneys. Such foods offer ideal protection
from a deficiency of qi and should be eaten frequently by
vegetarians.

Yet too much of the sweet-warm taste—for example,
in the form of fried meat—depletes the fluids of the
kidneys through the control cycle. This can lead to heat
illnesses and a yin deficiency of the kidneys, with hair loss,
bone decalcification, and dental problems.

Nutrition for Children

When it comes to nutrition for children, earth foods should
make up the largest portion of their diet. Children need
these sweet-tasting foods, because they particularly nourish
and develop the body. In addition, sweet foods have a moistening and relaxing effect. By nature, children have a lot of
qi and yang so that they can grow fast. Sweet foods provide
the balance for this by moistening and thus cooling. When
children get too little sweet food, they become extremely
restless and may also develop a craving for sweets. Of
course, sugar is as bad for children as it is for adults. But it
is virtually impossible to keep children entirely away from
sugar, unless you live on an isolated island.

The best way to nourish children in a healthy,
balanced, and mostly sugar-free way is to feed them earth
foods in any form. Small children do not need changes
constantly. Give them carrots with pumpkin, and the next
day pumpkin with carrots. Toddlers normally will not

mind. Cook stewed fruits, sweet soufflès, polenta, and millet, and your children will get everything they need. If they do not want to eat these things, try adding some organic butter, sesame oil, or other cold-pressed oils, which will also make the foods more nutritious.

Forgo tropical fruits and milk products as long as possible. One reason children have colds so often is because it is easier, for example, to give them cottage cheese or yogurt with bananas than cooking millet, especially in view of the fact that the former is normally rated so highly from the perspective of nutrition. From the point of view of Chinese medicine, however, cottage cheese or yogurt and bananas have a decidedly cooling and mucus-building energetic effect, and so should be avoided.

Metal

The small yin of the metal element drives away the yang forces, such as the strong heat of the summer. The increase in the yin forces, which are turned downward and inward, causes the juices of the plant world in the fall to retreat into the roots and the earth, drying out the leaves. In the fall, the forces of nature return to their origins.

Trust in the potential of the endless space that surrounds us, which is the domain of our origins, and which contains everything and makes everything possible, is the basis for the initial trust manifested in people with a strong metal element. From this comes the ability to persevere and to build up, on a material level, our lives. Holding one's own, paired with fairness, and an alert mind, along with active compassion, are the positive features of the metal phase, when life experience has sharpened the mind and secured one's existence.

The lungs and the large intestine, white, dryness, and the pungent taste are allocated to the metal element.

The Lungs and the Large Intestine

Aside from the earth organs, the lungs are the most important source for producing postnatal qi. The lungs extract qi from the air we breathe, which mixes in the Upper Burner with the nutrition qi of the spleen, and from there nourishes the entire organism.

The lungs control the functions of the skin: the opening and the closing of pores, the secretion of sweat, the moisture content, and thus the skin's elasticity. A major task of the lungs is to provide resistance energy, or "wei qi," which penetrates and enfolds the entire body. Resistance energy protects us from all disturbing influences of a climatic or chemical nature and from radiation. Westerners generally have a hard time accepting this, but for the Chinese it goes without saying that wei qi is what protects us from all accidents and conflicts, as they reflect a weakness of resistance qi.

The lungs are situated in the Upper Burner, together with the heart, the seat of the spirit. The condition of the lungs has a great deal to do with the condition of our psyche and our mental state. Accidents, illnesses, and conflicts—actually every form of suffering people experience—have their origins in the negative impressions in the spirit and the mind, which people have accumulated there through damaging deeds, words, and thoughts concerning themselves and others. The results are a weakness of the resistance energy and the difficult experiences that this brings forth. On the other hand, positive impressions gather in the mind because of useful and loving deeds, words, and thoughts, and lead to happy experiences, as well as to internal and external wealth. These connections clarify the close relationship and interaction between body and mind, which are taken into consideration in a holistic way of thinking. It is not by chance that Western medicine often considers many lung diseases and illnesses of the large intestine to have a psychosomatic component.

The lungs control the *skin,* the place of direct contact that connects us to the environment and to other people. The increase of skin disorders in the West is not only caused by the pollution of the environment through radiation and toxins and by incorrect nutrition and eating habits but also to a large extent by the relationship and communication problems in these fast-paced, stressful times.

The nose and the sense of smell are also subject to the control function of the lungs. Aromatherapy, which works with pure essential oils from plants, is based on the effect of fragrances on the body and the psyche. These essences are a real gift of nature and a wonderful balance for many of the damaging influences today.

Skin diseases such as neurodermatitis and many skin allergies are caused by functional disturbances of the lungs and the liver. In all such cases, it is important to elicit the causes of the problem thoroughly and to change one's diet. A strict diet with suitable grains and vegetables in many cases can detoxify and harmonize the organism, reducing or curing the problem. With children, avoiding milk products, white sugar, and pork has often shown to be beneficial in cases of neurodermatitis.

The large intestine has the task of detoxifying the body. The Chinese say, "Whatever the large intestine does not discharge must be discharged by the skin." Skin impurities and acne are the result of damp heat in the large intestine, caused by incorrect nutritional habits, but especially by consuming milk products and sugar, which create an ideal basis in the intestine for the growth of bacteria. In all cases of skin impurities, brown rice is the ideal remedy for detoxifying the large intestine.

In Chinese medicine, there are several causes for *constipation*. One has to do with a sluggishness of the large intestine due to a qi deficiency of the spleen and the lungs. This weakness can be found frequently in older people. When the lungs are weak, breathing becomes superficial. But deep breathing is necessary to maintain the proper functioning of the large intestine. Constipation is the result of weak breathing when the stool is somewhat soft and light-colored. Physical exercises and breathing therapy, combined with food rich in qi, are the best remedies in this case.

Another form of constipation takes place with a hard, dark stool. It occurs when the fluids of the large intestine have dried out. The causes of this can be consuming foods with a drying effect and stagnation of liver qi. Emotional tension, stress, and time pressure cause the qi of the liver to stagnate, and intestinal movement becomes sluggish. Food pulp remains too long in the intestine, becoming dry and hard. In this situation, it is important to moisten the large intestine and to relax the liver. For both, brown rice, juicy vegetables, and stewed fruits are recommended, along with physical movement.

Stomach heat, which leads to ravenous hunger, so that frequently large quantities of food are consumed, can also cause dry constipation in the long run, as the heat in the stomach promotes dryness in the large intestine.

Emotions and Mental Analogies

Initial trust—trust in the positive possibilities of our own existence—develops in a baby when it feels secure, cared for, and loved. These are all requirements for the infant to be able to develop and grow. Pleasant experiences cause, on all levels, a process of healthy expansion and development. On the physical level, openness and the state of being relaxed are the basis for the qi to be able to flow harmoniously and for all organs to be supplied in a balanced manner. On the emotional and mental levels, being able to open up and let go is the foundation for positive relationships and for mental and spiritual growth.

Illness and emotional suffering always go hand in hand with tightness, stagnation, conditions of fullness or emptiness, and muscular armor.

Spaciousness and expansion are analogies of the metal element. The realization of the true nature of space, the experience whereby we perceive that the spirit is boundless and cannot be destroyed, counteracts existential insecurity, fear, and the dependency on the body, and is a source of unconditional joy.

Space and expansion are essential for a healthy functioning of the lungs. When people are burdened emotionally, or when they suffer from fear and sadness, breathing becomes shallow and the upper body hangs. When people feel attacked, or when they can't deal with their own aggressions, the shoulders and the upper body are tense, which constricts the capacity of the lungs. Persistent sadness causes a qi weakness of the lungs; hurt and feelings regarding injustice lead to suppressed rage. Such emotions disturb the metal element and can cause, even in children, lung diseases and illnesses of the large intestine.

In Europe, the lung diseases that were widespread

after the Second World War were only partially caused by malnutrition. Emotional causes also played a large role; there was a great deal of existential fear and sadness regarding the loss of loved ones. Worry about the future and about one's existence also contributes to the development of lung diseases in many cases. Conversely, sadness and insecurity may come about when the lungs are damaged by external influences.

Dryness

Dryness damages the lungs and the large intestine in particular. Not only are we affected by overly dry climates but also by dry indoor air. The air in many workplaces is often a problem because of toxic fumes from furniture, wall-to-wall carpets, and wall paints but also because of its dryness. Yet overly dry indoor air can be corrected so easily: Simply put a container of water on the radiator, as was done in the old days, or install a fountain.

Have you ever been in a Chinese restaurant without an aquarium or a fountain? Probably not, and for a very good reason: Aside from humidifying the air, running water in rooms keeps the qi moving and, through this, is believed to bring money. You are welcome to dismiss this as superstition, but if you are ever in Hong Kong look around inside the large banks. In one after another, you'll see oversized fountains decorating the interior, installed on the advice of feng-shui consultants (feng shui is the practice of directing the qi movement in rooms for beneficial effects).

Try it yourself: Place a small fountain in your workroom, and let it run permanently. However, under no circumstances should you shut it off during the night;

otherwise, the qi will stagnate. If you should be offered a raise or win the lottery afterward, you may give half of it to me.

The Pungent Taste

All pungent vegetables such as onions, radishes, and leeks are primarily white. Other vegetables like comfrey, celery, and cauliflower are also white, meaning they have a portion of the metal element, but due to their mild taste are allocated to the earth element.

The pungent taste opens the pores of the body, moves the qi to the outside, and dissolves stagnation. Most pungent foods are either pungent-warm or pungent-hot; only a few are pungent-neutral or pungent-refreshing. The pungent-warm taste plays an important role in the treatment of cold illnesses. As soon as the cold penetrates the body, it closes the pores. In order to drive away the cold, the pores must be opened, which takes place through sweating. The pungent-warm taste induces sweat and is heating. Ginger tea and hot alcohol such as hot spicy wine are the right remedies when you feel a head cold coming on. Then, a rice dish with leeks, onions, and pungent spices is advised, as this affects the lungs and thus strengthens the body's resistance.

The pungent-warm taste moves the qi in the body upward, which is a desirable effect when people feel down or sad. Unfortunately, this result is frequently the initial cause for alcoholism as well. *Alcohol* dissolves the qi stagnation of the liver, as well as the tense frustration that goes along with it. If the cause for the frustration is not eliminated, however, turning to alcohol can become a habit. The relaxing effect of the pungent taste dissipates not only the bad mood but also the body's qi at the same time. This is the reason people often feel completely depleted after an alcoholic binge.

Pungent-warm foods are the best protection from cold weather in the winter. They strengthen the lungs, which are challenged a great deal during the flu season. By means of the generative cycle, they have a positive effect on the yang of the kidneys. In addition, they set the resistance qi, the overall flow of qi in the body, and the blood flow in motion, as they are always slowed down when it is cold.

The correct amount of pungent-warm foods is crucial. Too much pungent-warm taste in the form of alcohol or pungent spices diffuses the qi and overheats the liver and the gallbladder in particular by means of the control cycle. Garlic, alcohol, and pungent food, when consumed by people who already suffer from liver heat and inner tension, can lead to irritability and muscular tension. In addition, eye problems such as burning or itching can occur. A heat condition in the lungs can develop as well, and this leads to coughing. The kidneys become dry, resulting in hyperactivity and excessive sexual desire, which should not be confused with sexual potency. The heat brings about dryness in the large intestine, causing constipation. Pungent foods can also raise blood pressure, so if you already have high blood pressure, eat these foods with caution.

When the lungs are overly moist and produce a lot of light-colored mucus, foods with a bitter-warm taste are the right remedy. Grain coffee, thyme tea, buckwheat, and toasted millet dry out the dampness. Conversely, when done to excess, consuming bitter-warm stimulants such as coffee, black tea, and red wine, as well as smoking cigarettes, dry out the lungs and then the skin as well. Chronic dryness of the lungs is one of the causes of cancer and skin diseases. Pungent-refreshing foods—primarily brown rice, but also radishes, kohlrabi, and watercress—ensure that the lungs are moistened, and produce beautiful, youthful skin. Asparagus has the same effect. Asparagus is sweet (earth), bitter (fire), and white (metal). Use it as frequently as you can when it is in season, because asparagus is a real fountain of youth for the skin.

In cases of constipation with hard stool, it's helpful to eat steamed radishes with some butter and salt. Or, radish juice can be bought at the health-food store; have 1 to 2 tablespoons after meals.

Brown rice and the refreshing vegetables have a relaxing, fluid-building effect on the liver and the gall-bladder by means of the control cycle. Thus, the fluids of the kidneys are restored through the generative cycle.

Water

The water element is associated with the great yin of the winter. Now all movement is directed downward and inward. Qi and fluids retreat to the farthest inside places, concentrating in the earth and in seeds and roots. In the winter, yin, cold, and darkness predominate.

The water element stands for the twilight years and old age, as well as for the wise person whose highest virtue is modesty, as he or she has realized the transitory nature of all things and of human existence.

In Chinese paintings, we often see large mountains and in-between very small people, just the way things actually are. In European paintings, in comparison, we find, for example, a very large hunter in the foreground, the stag somewhat smaller behind him, and the forest and the mountains behind it very small way in the background.

The more our view is directed to the outside, the smaller the world seems to us and the larger we perceive ourselves—this is an illusion normally maintained all our lives. But when the mind is inner-directed and at peace, there is the necessary distance from the busyness of daily life, which gives us a more realistic way of looking at things. In addition, the dislike and the denial in the West of everything that has to do with death undermine our view of the world, causing us to perceive ourselves as the center of the universe and as immortal.

The mind can be compared to the eye: The eye looks to the outside but does not perceive itself doing this. In Buddhist meditation, where the focus is inside, we come to realize that the observer and that being observed, as well as the act of observing, are one. Also, we soon see the value of the mind being left to rest in its natural state, which is peace, without rejecting or desiring anything. This is the path toward realizing our internal wealth, active compassion, and wisdom.

The lotus flower, whose beauty and purity only unfold in swampy, cloudy water, is a symbol for the transformation of such feelings as greed and rage into wisdom, the highest feature of the water element. Water always takes the easiest path and flows downward into the depths. But through its persistent flow, it moves mountains. Reflection, seeing behind things, perseverance, and persistence are yin aspects of the water element. True fearlessness, which comes about when we realize that something in ourselves is timeless and cannot be destroyed, is a yang aspect of the water element.

The kidneys and the bladder, the colors blue and black, the climatic factor of coldness, and the salty taste are allocated to the water element.

The Kidneys and the Bladder

People with strong kidneys, the primary organ associated with the water element, are often granted courage, resolution, adamant willpower, success, and a long life. The kidneys are the storehouse for prenatal qi. Surplus qi, the result of gaining postnatal qi, is stored in the kidneys as well. The kidneys control the bones, the bone marrow, the brain, the central nervous system, the teeth, and the hair on our head, as well as the sense of hearing and the ears. They have the greatest influence on the sexual domain— on fertility, seminal power, potency, and libido. The genetic predisposition and the constitution of the newborn child depend on the kidney strength of the parents. Traditionally, Chinese parents prepare for the conceiving of a child for two years by strengthening their spleen and kidney qi through diet and physical exercises.

The yang aspects of the kidneys are qi and warmth. Should they be weakened, people have cold feet, knees, and hips, and a cold posterior. They also suffer from back pain early in the morning, which improves through movement after getting up. They tend to urinate frequently and have the need to urinate during the night. A weak libido and infertility are other signs they exhibit. In addition, they feel weak generally and sometimes anxious and depressed. Often they experience a craving for coffee or Coke to overcome their exhaustion.

Do you remember the image of the flaring kidney fire in the Lower Burner, which rises up to the earth organs and to the Upper Burner? When the fire element is too weak, the spleen, the stomach, the heart, and the lungs are not warmed sufficiently anymore, and a deficiency of qi and coldness are the result. Conversely, if the fire element gets out of control should there be a fluid deficiency in the kidneys, an internal feeling of heat, restlessness, sleep disorders, nervousness, a low tolerance of stress, and a lack of perseverance can develop. At night, the person breaks out in a sweat and is aware of having hot soles of the feet. Disorders that go hand in hand with a substance deficiency, such as osteoporosis (bone decalcification), also result.

Aside from storing qi, the kidneys reserve fluids. If too little fluid is produced, a yin deficiency can develop in the kidneys. This can spread to other organs over the course of time, especially to the liver, the stomach, or the heart.

The excretory function of the bladder depends essentially on a healthy functioning of the kidneys. The earlier described bladder infection as a result of heart fire is the exception to this. Chronic bladder infections are quite common today in women. The cause for the aforementioned type of bladder infection was time pressure and stress. The other cause of bladder infections is coldness that penetrates from the outside, which is intensified when there is a kidney-yang weakness.

Emotions and Mental Analogies

In Eastern psychology, there are different kinds of fear. I want to mention two here: on the one hand, the fearful insecurity concomitant with a yang weakness of the kidneys and, on the other, the fear of repercussions from unleashing aversion and rage into the world.

Fearful insecurity, or feelings of anxiety, when there is a kidney-yang weakness, results from overall feebleness and exhaustion. When the yang force of the kidneys is strong, however, we have the will and the courage to forcefully set about our life with all of its challenges and to face the difficulties.

Avoiding responsibility, capitulating, and not standing up for yourself or for others are patterns of behavior associated with a kidney-yang weakness. But to hold your own means to face the tasks and the conflicts of life. Withdrawing from the start is cowardly and indicates most of the time that we put the responsibility onto someone else. Courage, on the other hand, is the readiness to accept responsibility for something and to fight for what we believe in. You strengthen your own powers of resistance and the yang of the kidneys by facing facts, developing some brazenness, and showing guts. Should you then come to realize that your "opponent" has the better argument, you can retreat, without losing face, and gratefully admit that you have learnt something.

Constantly seeking confrontation in order to prove to yourself and to others that you are superior in some way, however, suggests that you actually feel less than equal. This confrontational attitude is an aspect of "macho" behavior that women exhibit nowadays just as frequently as men do. The wise Chinese saying, "The person who does not fight wins in reality," corresponds to the provident way the Chinese lead their lives. They strengthen themselves from the start—whether on the health front or that of their personality—in order to be armed in the event of an attack, so that the attack rebounds. The equanimity and the lack of defensiveness with which some people handle criticism, seeing it as an opportunity for personal growth rather than an attack, is a manifestation of a type of strength achieved by cultivating inner calmness. A strong center, which nourishes the organism, is extremely helpful here. What's more, the satiated feeling of a well-filled belly—as banal as this may seem—is an excellent basis for a healthy resistance, on both the physical level and the level of the psyche.

The basis for the second kind of fear is rage. When we permit ourselves again and again to be overcome by rage, envy, or dislike, inner heat develops in the area of the liver and the gallbladder, and then we feel burnt out and empty. Sending negativity out into the world eventually leads to a state of feeling insecure and threatened, and we think we have to arm ourselves against the world. Then, it is no wonder that we repeatedly find reasons for getting agitated or annoyed. In terms of the root cause, it can be assumed that this lack of trust in the world was developed to some degree already in childhood.

In order to overcome this second type of fear and to find our own inner strength, it is necessary to give up our hostile attitudes. To succeed in this, we must be willing to see that, aside from our own rigid views, say, regarding what we dislike about another person, there are other ways of looking at things. This in turn requires that we take our own feelings less seriously. One moment, when we are happy, everybody is nice; but should our mood shift a minute later, we can't see anything good about anyone. Is it really the world that executes these gymnastics? Or is it rather our own mind that suddenly makes enemies out of friends and misleads us into destroying trust in a few minutes of rage? Anyone who goes through life in a sour mood finds reasons everywhere that support this. By contrast, anyone who looks kindly into the world sees reasons to be joyful and benevolent. Therefore, it's important not to take those moments where you are wearing your dark pair of glasses so seriously.

In order to master negative, aggressive habits, it's helpful to realize that emotions are often a very shaky affair and that they draw their strength mainly from the fact that we identify with them so strongly and take them so seriously. If we succeeded only once in seeing clearly the phenomenon that occurs when there is a storm—in observing the clouds and the rain and then the sun shining again—the year would soon have more sunny days.

This is not the same as repressing. On the contrary, it is a matter of identifying the enemy, instead of being out there, as your own rage or envy, and then perhaps investing this energy into some kind of meaningful work that you have postponed for a long time. Maybe you are thinking, this is easier said than done. You are right, but it works. Try it.

When you are once again close to smashing your expensive Chinese vase, sit down and fold your hands in your lap. Close your eyes. You are on the right track if what you are experiencing is just as suspenseful as watching the eruption of a volcano. First, you see only fire. Now try to find out where the center of the fire is: in your head, in your chest, in your feet? Take time, and look. The fire will become weaker and weaker, and soon you will be able to breathe again. A sense of spaciousness returns. The fire has disappeared. How do you feel now? Probably very good—and not only because the vase is still intact.

Regarding the investment of energy in work, this also involves looking within. Just as we should eat foods that we like, that appeal to us, we should do work that we like, that resonates with who we are.

Once you experience time and again how rage develops and dissipates, it will lose its strength and power over you. An inner strength is the result.

It takes courage and a certain degree of inner stability to be able to give yourself over to such inner experiences when you are filled with rage. In these cases, it might be advisable to see a counselor or a therapist, in order to have your first experiences with visualization in a protected environment. It should be the goal of therapy to uncover the loving, creative parts of a person. This holds true in general when we deal with people. If we focus our attention on the positive qualities of others, we see people more often in light of their potential; if we look at the imperfections, we see bunglers everywhere. Moreover, if we see a friend in other people, we feel at home in the large human family and do not need to be afraid.

How to Strengthen the Kidneys

Fear, as well as aggression, are protective mechanisms. But we need to have a healthy dose of courage and confidence in order to strengthen the kidneys. Risk something. Jump over a brook in the summer, even if you are not sure whether or not you will land safely on the other side. Speak to a person with whom you have wanted to be in contact forever but didn't dare. What can happen? If you are rejected, at least you will know where you stand. And a positive reaction will bolster your self-confidence.

What makes people successful? They dare to do things that others don't dare to do. Some are courageous and persevering by nature, meaning they have good kidneys. Others may have overcome their fears, fought their dislikes, and rechanneled their aggressions time and time again, and through that strengthened their self-confidence, and thus their kidneys. Giving in to anxiety and passivity not only makes for a boring life but also is detrimental to the kidneys. The kidneys need a certain amount of tension in daily life and in love relationships. The best kidney medicine is sexual pleasure, closeness, and tenderness, on the basis of a good relationship.

Cold Weather

Heat, which can manifest as a fever, a bladder infection, or a kidney infection, normally develops in the body as a reaction to cold weather, the climatic factor allocated to the water element. A qi or yang deficiency, or, said differently, a resistance weakness, is the predisposition whereby coldness can penetrate into the body. Qi and warmth are the protective shields against external coldness, and they are produced by two factors: movement and nutrition. A lack of movement can be counteracted relatively well with warming food. A lack of qi or yang, on the other hand, cannot be balanced anymore through movement when a person keeps eating unbalanced food.

Especially if you already suffer from coldness or if you easily become cold, you should protect yourself from cold weather through appropriate clothing. Cold penetrates through the feet, to the lower-back and genital area, into the organism, so keeping the feet and the back warm is a good precaution. Of course, this doesn't eliminate the yang deficiency and the sensitivity to coldness. For this, it is necessary to build up the qi and the yang again through neutral and warming foods.

The Salty Taste

Black foods such as seaweed and black soybeans are allocated to the water element, as are all kinds of seafood and legumes, because they have an energetic effect on the kidneys.

The water element's salty taste has laxative, mucus-dissolving, and emollient effects. In small quantities, it increases the bodily fluids and combines them in the right places. Too much salt has the exact opposite effect: The body dries out and hardens, and mental attitudes stiffen as well.

People who eat very salty food need a counterbalance in order to remoisten the body. They do this with sweet food. By means of the generative cycle, the lack of dampness of the kidney yin, due to too much salt, affects the liver and the gallbladder. Internal tension and emotional irritability are the result. As the sweet taste relaxes, the nutritional habits of many people are determined by alternating extremely sweet and salty foods; for example, they may eat chocolate during the day and potato chips in the evening.

Salt and alcohol are another strange pair. At first, the fluids in the alcoholic beverage replenish the dampness that was extracted due to too much salt. But then the surplus salt is excreted together with the fluids. However, alcohol later has a drying-out effect, even in small quantities. In addition, alcohol loosens emotional tensions sometimes to such a degree that the person becomes sentimental and emotionally unstable, and this has to be counteracted through an artificial hardening with salt. In order to break out of this vicious cycle, one's salt consumption should be restricted at first. Then, it is easier to get a grip on the craving for alcohol and for sweets.

Sausage and cold cuts, cheese, and even bread often contain a lot of hidden salt. If you are used to salt, dishes with little salt taste bland at the beginning. But if you forgo strongly salted food for a while, the sense of taste quickly gets used to food low in salt. Food that tasted good before seems too salty now.

Salt is cold in terms of its thermal effect. However, through its drying influence, it causes a deficiency of yin, so heat symptoms in the kidneys, the liver, the gallbladder, and, through the control cycle, the heart can develop.

All fish and seafood belong to the water element. In general, it can be said that saltwater fish are warming and freshwater fish neutral. Shrimp has a warm thermal effect. Crab, seaweed, mussels, and caviar, on the other hand, are considered cold.

Legumes are refreshing or neutral, bean sprouts cold. Salty-warm foods strengthen the yang of the kidneys, from which the Middle and Upper Burners profit. Legumes are a nourishing food that strengthens qi. Salty-refreshing food builds up the fluids of the kidneys and of the entire organism. Salty-cold seaweed protects us from excessive kidney fire and from heart heat by means of the control cycle. Seaweed is an important supplier of many minerals as well.

The Role of Drinking Water

Mineral water has salty-cold properties. Some brands of mineral water are so high in sodium that they are almost undrinkable. If you frequently add salt to food, because the food tastes too bland without it, check the sodium content of the mineral water you drink normally. If it is relatively high, it's no wonder that you often reach for the saltshaker.

People often ask me what they should drink in order to consume the daily requirement of 3 quarts, or liters, of liquid. This rule is nonsense, as far as I'm concerned, despite being so widespread. Many people force themselves to drink large quantities of high-sodium mineral water even though they are not thirsty at all, because they are under the impression that this is good for them. Of course, we all need to consume liquids, but exactly how much is an individual matter.

If you eat meat, sausage, or smoked food, you will easily drink 3 quarts, or liters, of fluids per day, because you will be very thirsty. However, if vegetables, salad, and fruits are a large portion of your diet, 3 cups of herbal tea can be sufficient. In cases of a spleen weakness with dampness, the need to drink is minimal, because the transformation of what is drunk into the body's own fluids is reduced a great deal. Through the decreased thirst, the body protects itself from additional strain from fluids. A yin or blood deficiency also lessens the need to drink. In such a case, we are thirsty and the body is lacking fluids, but we disregard this. Now, it's a good idea to have a thermos with a hot beverage at hand and to drink little sips throughout the day.

For building up bodily fluids, aside from drinking liquids it is crucial to eat juicy, briefly cooked vegetables and stewed fruits. If you replenish your fluids this way, not only will you be supplying the body with water but also with vital nutrients, which when part of whole food—in contrast to extracts—can be well metabolized. This is probably not the case, however, with artificially enriched mineral water.

Anyone who believes that excess fluids are simply excreted, without putting strain on the body, errs. In fact, excess fluids put pressure on the kidneys, because they must filter out and excrete everything that is drunk. In addition, the high mineral content in mineral water cannot be utilized in the body and is a strain. Drinking an excessive amount of cold beverages eventually leads to a weakness of the yang in the kidneys. In some places where carrying around a large bottle of spring water has almost become fashionable, even young people are having problems with incontinence. This symptom of a kidney-yang weakness in the past was seen only in the elderly or in conjunction with a kidney disease.

Tap water, if derived from wells, contains exactly the right portion of minerals. Insecticides, pesticides, and chlorine are the main problems when it comes to water pollution. You can protect yourself from this by using a water filter. But you should be aware that most appliances that remove the lime at the same time filter out most of the minerals, which of course is not their purpose. There are also devices that add carbonic acid to the filtered water, so that the water will have that bubbly effect.

Love and Sexuality

The Yellow Emperor said to the young peasant woman: "I lost my vital energy, and I have fallen out of harmony. There is no joy anymore in my heart. My body is exhausted and has become sickly. What shall I do?"

The young woman answered: "The cause of men's weakness lies solely in their misuse of the male-female relationship. Women, on the other hand, are superior to men in this respect, just as water is superior when it extinguishes fire. If you understand this and apply it correctly, you will resemble the cooking pots on the tripods in which the five types of taste are blended harmoniously so that a delicious soup made of meat and vegetables is created. Anyone who knows about the ways of the female and male elements participates in the five pleasures; anyone who does not know about them and does not respect them will shorten his life. What pleasures and delights could be discovered and experienced! Who would not pay attention to this?"

—From *Fang Chung Shu* (*The Chinese Art of Love*)

Unfortunately, the young woman was not specific when she made reference to the five pleasures. Yet anyone can easily imagine the pleasures and delights that can be discovered and experienced when yin and yang are united. But what did the young woman mean when she said that women are superior to men? If you think that the Taoists were the predecessors of today's feminists, you are sadly mistaken.

In ancient China, people believed that men lose more vital energy through ejaculation during the act of making love than women do through their orgasm, and this made women superior to men. In addition, it was assumed that the man's semen nourished the woman energetically. But the reverse was also believed to be true—that a woman with a strong yin nourished the man, as long as he ejaculated as little as possible.

Ideally, the goal of sexual union should be to increase the vital energy of both the man and the woman. This happens automatically through the exchange of fluids and qi during intercourse, as long as other factors do not interfere, such as a lack of love between the partners and having sexual relations before both partners are ready.

It has been known from time immemorial in China that the woman needs longer for the yang of her excitement to unfold, so it was the man's duty to hold back his yang, which he has available much sooner. Thus, for the man, it was a matter of course for him to curb his lust, so that his female partner would be ready, and then could reach her orgasm possibly several times, and so that he could preserve his semen, the life essence. Forgoing ejaculation was, in addition, a process whereby the man could have the greatest pleasures and the most intense orgasms without losing his semen. In ancient China, it was also the custom for wealthy old men to be supplied with very young, healthy women, in order to renew their vital energies. However, the noblest goal of the sexual union was to refine the life essence (jing) to such a degree that it could rise in the organism, in order to nourish the spirit and thus serve one's spiritual development.

The following description is certainly only a very limited excerpt from the abundance of material from the

Chinese concerning the energetic and healing effects of the sexual union.

"When she (the woman) nourishes the female element with the help of the male element, a myriad of illnesses are driven away; her complexion will glow, her skin becomes smooth and clear, and years go by without her showing any signs of aging. When the woman pursues this course steadfastly and has intercourse frequently with men, she will not feel hunger even when she has not eaten for nine days."

It is understood that the above statements refer to a very high level of physical love. The sexual union, when part of meditative exercises, was a means to strengthen vital energy, in order to achieve heightened awareness and health. At this high level of physical love, the partners interact with each other sensibly and consciously, and every facet of lovemaking is allowed to reach the highest ecstasy.

Even today Taoists believe that the "jade shaft" and the "jade grotto" should remain united for a while following the climax, so that the seminal fluids and the fluids of the vagina can mix with each other. The exchange of the two is thought to strengthen the health and the vitality of the lovers.

Looked at energetically, a woman can develop her female potential increasingly through fulfilled sexuality. She becomes more loving while also more self-composed. At the same time, she has the possibility of taking on the strong sides of her partner. If a woman is rather shy and introverted, she can learn to overcome her reserve through an intimate, loving relationship with a man who makes contact easily with people. Conversely, a guy with rough edges will sooner or later develop a certain degree of friendliness and sensitivity through the inspiration of a gentle female partner. The energetic exchange through fulfilled sexuality is one of the most secret, wonderful gifts of love. It reveals itself most when both partners not only express what they want sexually but are also more concerned with the pleasure of their lover than with their own satisfaction.

Causes of Sexual Problems

Prenatal qi and postnatal qi, which is produced from nutrition and from the air we breathe, are stored in the kidneys. Together, they form the basis for the yang (fire) and the yin (fluids) of the kidneys. Kidney fire is the foundation for overall strength and self-confidence, as well as for erotic charisma, sexual potency, and libido. The fluids of the kidneys serve as the basis for fertility and perseverance, as well as for the ability to show sympathetic understanding, to experience closeness and tenderness, and to open and surrender oneself.

From the Western point of view, sexual disorders have to do with actual problems with one's spouse or partner, earlier traumatic experiences, being raised in a way that was hostile toward sexuality, or suppressed childhood abuse. As long as the disorder is within the realm of a neurosis, psychotherapy is the recommended form of treatment.

Traditional Chinese medicine deals with sexual disorders in a fundamentally different manner. For one thing, a constellation of completely different causes is considered: the person's innate constitution, the relationship to the parents, and the influence of the social environment, in addition to nutrition and climatic conditions. What's more, it is believed that disturbing factors from childhood do not express themselves in emotional or sexual problems alone, but always on an organic and energetic level as well. It can also be said that negative influences on our organs like external coldness and cooling foods also trigger emotional and sexual problems. On the basis of this holistic view, sexual disorders demand treatment on an organic-energetic level as well as on the level of the psyche.

Every organic imbalance affects the psyche, the ability to love, and one's sexuality. But the greater imbalance there is, especially in the kidneys and the heart, the more one's sexuality is impaired.

When Kidney Fire Stops Burning

Impotence in men and inability to reach orgasm in women, of course, are serious problems in any love relationship, and are often treated through psychotherapy. Yet these problems are less common than the creeping love-killer: the lack of desire. When the periods between having sex become longer and longer, not because of difficulties with impotence or reaching orgasm, but simply because the partners do not feel like it, what is the matter? What should be done, for example, if the man still desires the woman, but she is always tired and simply does not feel any desire? Or if the woman has been wooing her partner for weeks, but he, despite all his love for her, can't forget about his work? What are the reasons why two people who love each other no longer have any desire to make love?

Nowadays many people seem to be preoccupied with their own problems to the extent that they have nothing left for the other person. When one person in a relationship is overly needy, problems in the relationship are also bound to develop. In addition, if people are overly critical of themselves—for example, when a woman sees her reflection in the mirror and feels it doesn't measure up to the current feminine ideal—they may feel they have little to offer. In reality, every person has a lot to give. But our problem is that we often do not focus on our internal wealth but instead on our internal poverty. Egocentrism, neediness, and a lack of self-esteem all are love-killers.

From the viewpoint of TCM, lack of sexual desire is not relegated to the psychological realm alone. Chinese medicine also looks at the energetic triggers. The foremost cause of lack of sexual interest (and physical exhaustion) is a deficiency of yang in the kidneys. The second probable cause is liver qi stagnation, which was explained in the section on the wood element, together with recommendations on to how to deal with it.

Generally, men are not as affected by a yang weakness of the kidneys as women are, because their kidney fire is stronger constitutionally. But physical, emotional, and mental stress, as well as sweets, qi-less foods, and ice-cold beverages create a strong tendency for this in men too. Because women have more yin (blood and fluids) but less yang (qi and warmth), they tend to suffer more from coldness and being overweight. Their concern with keeping their weight down often entices them to prefer cooling foods such as yogurt, uncooked food, and tropical fruits. In general, women tend to eat more cooling foods like salads, fruits, and milk products, and to reject warming foods like meat (usually favored by men) mostly because of their awareness of the current trends in nutrition. What's more, women are often extremely overburdened when they have a job in addition to a family.

Strong cravings for sweets and sugar are a result of a

spleen qi weakness. Because the kidney fire must warm the Middle Burner (the spleen), it is also affected in the long run when there is a spleen weakness. In addition, refined sugar lowers the yang of the kidneys through the control cycle, so it is the number-one love-killer among the foods. The high consumption of sweets nowadays is one of the main causes of decreased libido and problems with impotence.

When the culprit is mainly mistakes in nutrition, the situation can be reversed through correct nutrition that strengthens the yang of the kidneys. If you want to fan the flames of desire, you can produce heat with these delicious dishes:

- Lamb or beef marinated in red wine; beef broth with leeks; beef with horseradish; mutton with garlic; pheasant, venison, or wild boar; chicken soup with spring onions and curry; chicken sautéed in butter with a lot of fresh ginger and curry and enriched with sake (rice wine).
- Fresh salmon, tuna, eel, anchovies, and shrimp, fried, barbecued, and smoked, with roasted walnuts, cooked in wine, with clove powder.
- Leeks baked with goat cheese; pumpkin with thyme and a shot of vodka; fennel and carrots with red wine and chili.
- Roasted rice with spring onions and roasted pine nuts; roasted millet cooked in red wine; fresh corn with chili; polenta with roasted buckwheat; spelt with onions cooked in wheat beer.
- Stewed apples with cinnamon and cardamom, roasted walnuts, and honey; baked apricots with rum raisins.

@ Stay away from ice cream and salads, as well as lemonade, soft drinks, white wine, and beer. Instead, offer your lover a glass of really good full-bodied red wine or some hot sake.

Soon the ice will thaw, and where there was once disinterest will be a renewal of desire.

When the Fountain Runs Dry

People whose kidneys are lacking fluids experience a fear of closeness and tenderness. They may have developed an armor of restraint that prevents them from showing any spontaneous expression of their feelings, leaving their spouse or partner hoping in vain for any signs of affection or sympathetic understanding. These tendencies can be caused and intensified by liver qi stagnation. On the other hand, people whose kidneys are lacking yang do not have enough energetic tension, which causes impotence in a man and lack of desire and inability to reach orgasm in a woman. The lack of fluids leads to muscular overstrain and overstrain of the nerves, so that a man tends to ejaculate prematurely, thus carrying out the act of love fast and insensitively. Due to the increased tension and nervousness, the woman is not able to let go in experiencing desire and in reaching orgasm. Emotional blockages keep men and women from feeling deep and tender feelings, so the act of having sex is no longer much about bonding and giving and receiving pleasure, but merely becomes a way of releasing tensions.

Nervousness and tension are often the result of a misunderstood desire for intensity. People who mistake self-possession for boredom often stimulate themselves with coffee, Coke, red wine, or cigarettes. Internal tension, frequently the result of these drying stimulants, then leads people to believe that they are experiencing things with excitement and intensity. The increasing inability to truly feel things intensely pushes people more and more into external activities whose purpose is to stimulate, until possibly an illness stops them in their tracks or recurring disappointments in love relationships wake them up.

Meditative movement exercises, such as tai chi and qigong, or therapeutic bodywork, like bioenergetics, help to crack the armor concealing feelings and to bring once prohibited feelings to the surface. Now, better able to feel and express tenderness and closeness with their partner, the chase for external stimulants becomes unnecessary. Many of my colleagues who practice and teach tai chi have seen that the need for coffee and cigarettes also clearly diminishes.

In terms of nutrition, all bitter, drying foods—but especially coffee, black tea, red wine, and hot chocolate—should be avoided, and the bodily fluids should be replenished with vegetables, stewed fruits, fruit tea, grape juice, and grains like brown rice and wheat.

Coldness of the Heart

To love, without wanting to change your partner; to give of yourself, without leaving a little back door open; and to give your very best, without holding back—all reflect the harmony of the yin and yang of the heart. What is required here is a turning inside to be able to draw from the wealth of one's own feelings and from the breadth of the heart, in order to express joy, enthusiasm, and sincere tenderness to the outside.

A person with weak heart yang only rarely experiences intense feelings, is affected deeply by anything, or experiences boundless enthusiasm, and even more rarely expresses any of this. His or her spouse or partner often wishes in vain that he or she would make a loving gesture, say something complimentary, or play a more active role in their sex life. Yang weakness of the heart can also be the reason in a man for premature ejaculation and in a woman for the inability to reach orgasm. People who in their childhood didn't experience verbal or physical expressions of parental love, or who were taught that love and suffering go hand in hand, often have a hard time expressing the feelings of their heart.

Due to the yang weakness of the heart, the yin can rise excessively. In this situation, strong feelings are experienced as suffocating. Or, the person, unskilled in dealing with strong feelings, may express his or her passion uncontrollably. This, in the long run, will demand too much from any partner, even if hungry for love, so he or she will often end up reacting with rejection and anger.

Self-assurance and stability are necessary to corral the emotional chaos and to lead it toward a targeted, more moderate form of expression. Success in fields that do not require a great deal in terms of communication and organization—for example, creative or artistic activities—can help to develop self-confidence and create the necessary distance from the internal drama.

Without having to look to lack of parental warmth as a cause, the profit returns of the sweets industry are sufficient in showing that many people's hearts lie on ice, as too much sugar weakens the yang of the heart. The cravings for sweet food, as a result of a qi weakness of the spleen, are not recognized as such, so they are satisfied in the wrong manner. Satisfying the cravings for sweets with mild-sweet nutrition such as millet, beef, and carrots, on the other hand, not only strengthens the spleen but the heart as well. In contrast, sugar weakens the qi of the spleen. The heart is the "mother of the spleen." She engages her yang in order to support the weakened yang of the "child," eventually exhausting herself.

From the perspective of therapeutic nutrition, it is important to avoid sweet-cold foods like sugar, sweets, lemonade, soft drinks, ice cream, tropical fruits, and milk products. They all cool down the spleen and withdraw the yang from the heart. Sour-cold and salty-cold foods—such as yogurt, tomatoes, tropical fruits, uncooked food, white wine, fruit teas, and mineral water—have the same effect.

Yang-enhancing cooking methods like roasting, baking, and browning warm up the heart and reduce excess fluids. This is also the case with all neutral, warm, and qi-building foods, as well as those dishes that are recommended when there is a yang deficiency. Therefore, lamb or beef, in red wine, and toasted buckwheat are especially good to eat. Herbs that are helpful include thyme, oregano, and rosemary, as well as fenugreek powder, whose intense flavor takes full effect in stews and soups. Small quantities of coffee or grain coffee are also recommended, particularly when brought to a boil together with cardamom.

Rigid Love

Verbose, gushing declarations of love, sometimes with little internal foundation, are associated with people whose heart yin is weakened; the opposite holds true for those whose heart yang is weakened, meaning they hold back and express very little. Austerity and pedantry often keep such people from permitting themselves to express spontaneous feelings. Frequently this can be the result of a puritan upbringing, in which sexual feelings in particular but also fun and free-spirited enjoyment are attributed to the influence of the devil. The tendency toward religious rigidity can even be worsened with mental strain, lack of sleep, and drying foods and stimulants such as coffee, black tea, Coke, red wine, and cigarettes. Strong mental control has a way of blocking passionate feelings and the expression and buildup of sexual desire. This in turn could be the cause for sexual passivity and inability to reach orgasm in women and premature ejaculation in men.

Forms of creative stimulation and relaxation, with music or dancing in groups, for example, can help to loosen the internal rigidity and to develop more openness, expressiveness, spontaneity, and flexibility. When it comes to nutrition, bitter-drying foods and beverages like coffee, black tea, and red wine should be avoided. On the other hand, fluid-building, refreshing vegetables, grains, salads, and fruits, as well as rose-hip tea, prepared with yin-enhancing cooking methods, are known to strengthen the yin of the heart. In terms of overall lifestyle, try to avoid mental strain and reading for too long into the night. In contrast, sufficient sleep, walks, fresh air, and recuperation are all helpful.

Open meridians where the energy is flowing, as well as the overall elasticity of the body, are very important for a harmonious and intense love life, because they also open the heart. Achieving these features are some of the main goals of tai chi and qigong. Aside from these movement arts, the use of natural essential oils offers wonderful possibilities when it comes to shutting out the stresses of daily life and reaching more depth in feelings and sexual enjoyment. By having a relaxing and stimulating effect at the same time, fragrances can connect the contrasts of yin and yang in a way that cannot be imitated. Through the use of good-quality essential oils, a rough person can become more feeling and sensitive, someone who is prim can loosen up more and relax, a tentative person can become excited and let go, and a wallflower can blossom into a rose.

Effects of Processing, Freezing, and Microwaves

Sadly, in these fast-paced, stressful modern times, many people neglect preparing nutritious meals. Foods that are highly processed, frozen food, and foods defrosted or heated up in the microwave may make preparing dinner faster after a long day at work, but they extract a steep price when it comes to our health.

Over the course of the many years I have worked as a nutritional counselor, I have come across a wealth of information pointing to the fact that foods not produced by ecologically conscious companies, but by conventional industries, are damaging to our health. This holds true for the cultivation of vegetables and their subsequent processing, as well as for the breeding of animals for meat and milk products, and the breeding of fish. The quality of the waters from which we get our seafood also needs to be looked at, as does whether or not preservatives and synthetic substances for aroma and color are used.

Because it is difficult to investigate every product sold at conventional grocery stores, I recommend to everyone concerned about health to buy as much as possible at health-food stores or directly from the organic farmer. When I give people this advice, I am frequently confronted with the argument about price. Of course, high-quality food is initially more expensive than food of low quality, because the production and the storage are more costly. However, in the long run, basic foods like whole grains and legumes, which taste like what they are, are not expensive. This is because they produce a feeling of satiation, and in time not only will people's nutritional habits change but many things on which they formerly spent a lot of money will become unnecessary. People are often quite willing to spend a great deal of money, say, on furnishings for their home, clothes, cosmetics, and medicine. Yet when it comes to what they put into their bodies—and from what their organism develops newly again and again—they tend to hold back. Ironically, this ends up being uneconomical, not only because a healthy body requires less money for medical care but also because it is more attractive and needs less to keep it looking good.

Regarding the damaging effect of frozen food, to this day I can only base my claims on my own observations, as I have yet to find scientific research as proof. One idea, however, that has become fairly widespread has to do with shock freezing versus freezing very slowly. Now being applied in industry and more lately in people's homes, shock freezing is a method whereby the cell walls of foods are kept intact by means of very elaborate deep-freezing devices; in contrast, freezing foods very slowly destroys their cell walls.

From the point of view of TCM, through the process of deep-freezing food, the yin in food is increased, which means it becomes more cooling. It retains this feature even when it is defrosted and heated up or cooked. Therefore, when a food is subjected to deep freezing, we can assume this has an influence on the energetic effect of the food and thus on the ability of the organism to metabolize it (more about this follows the case studies). I am convinced that studies regarding the harmfulness of frozen food already exist and that it is merely a matter of time until they escape the lock and key of research institutes, where they now remain hidden because of the pressure of the food and electronics industries. This, in fact, has occurred with research concerning the effects on food from using the microwave.

Unfortunately, also certain foods sold at health-food stores are frozen in the process of being produced. For example, with dried fruit, a large portion of the fruit is kept frozen in storage until being dried. Rice is also partially frozen in order to prevent it from being infested by vermin. It is understandable that the health-food business wants to keep up with the wave of foods requiring little preparation and therefore is offering more and more frozen food as well. But by doing so, it violates its own rule: to offer high-quality nutrition. Food that was frozen at any point during its storage or production at least should be labeled accordingly.

Research regarding the damaging influences of microwaves—either from microwave ovens or foods treated with microwaves in their production—is somewhat more available. Yet independent research as well as widespread exposure of their results have been prevented in the past again and again from different sides. Therefore, to date not only has the size of studies still been relatively small but also the knowledge of the general public, when we consider how matter-of-factly and carelessly people use microwave ovens in daily life. The section on scientific knowledge concerning the dangers of the microwave spell out some interesting and alarming results from international research that goes back as far as 1942, and further details can be found in Appendix A.

Typical Cases from My Practice

But first I would like to present a brief account of my own experiences as a nutritional counselor that caused me already many years ago to start gathering information on this subject. Three cases from the beginning of my practice showed me especially clearly the negative effects of eating frozen food and food heated in the microwave oven.

The first case involves a middle-aged nutrition-conscious woman, in whom I diagnosed a highly pronounced qi weakness of the spleen with severe digestive problems, in addition to a kidney-yang deficiency and a resistance weakness. I was surprised by her condition, because her basic constitution was strong, her nutrition consisted of high-quality food bought exclusively at the health-food store, and she was an enthusiastic cook. Until then, I had observed a similar massive weakness of the qi of the Middle Burner only in people who either had a weak basic constitution or whose nutrition consisted of fast food, sweets, coffee, soft drinks, and so forth.

The solution to the riddle only emerged when I discussed with her the list of foods to be avoided and we came to the issue of frozen food. Completely astonished that something she was doing could be wrong, she told me that she was a busy, professional, single woman, and she bought everything she needed basically once a month in large quantities. Afterward, she stored everything—from bread to butter to vegetables—in a large freezer, from which she could take the food conveniently when she needed it, and then thaw it or thaw it and cook it. She also told me she did not own a microwave oven, because she was suspicious of it from the start, as, by the way, many other nutrition-conscious people have been.

Reluctantly, she agreed to use only fresh food for a while to see if it made any difference in her health. Just a couple of weeks into this new regime, she called me to report that she had given away her freezer, because her digestive problems had improved so much already and she felt much more vital.

The second case puzzled me at first, just as the first one did. Both partners of a married couple suffered from the same massive digestive problems and showed a strong kidney-yang weakness. In addition, the man had other illnesses. Ironically, they ran an organic farm in close proximity to relatives who also ran organic farms. Their food came almost entirely from the land. Every three months, they slaughtered on one of the farms and they baked bread. The bread and the meat ended up in a giant freezer, together with a large portion of the vegetable and fruit harvest. The foods were defrosted—without using a microwave oven—and eaten. I remember quite well how, after our consultation, I said good-bye to this couple with mixed feelings. I had shown them the advantages of methods of preserving food that did no harm, such as bottling and vacuuming, but I knew how much more time they would need having to make do without the freezer.

The third case has to do with a four-year-old girl whose mother brought her to see me. The child was the youngest of four siblings, and when she was born they had bought a microwave oven. Simply everything that this child had been fed as a baby and a toddler was heated up in the microwave. The mother had even frequently pumped her own milk and frozen it, so that the father could heat it up in the microwave and feed it to the baby. The woman came for help because her four-year-old, in contrast to the three older children, constantly had head colds and was tired, and she had suffered noticeably from bloating and abdominal cramps ever since she was very small. Her pale face and the dark rings under her eyes were striking in her appearance.

When I explained the connection between the child's weakness and the use of the microwave oven, the mother calculated back, because she also had begun to suffer from digestive problems, which had become more and more troublesome over time. She realized that her own digestive problems had begun almost precisely at the time when they had started to prepare meals in the microwave oven. The other children, who at least in their first years had been raised on fresh breast milk and conventionally heated food, had been able to cope with the microwave food better than the youngest one, probably because they had gotten a stable foundation from good childhood nutrition.

Of course, they immediately put the microwave oven in the basement, and the digestive problems of the mother and daughter soon became less severe, a sign that the spleen had recovered. But it is questionable whether the child will ever develop the constitution of her siblings.

This is my understanding as to why frozen food cannot be tolerated or digested: During slow freezing in particular, molecular structures and cell walls are changed and destroyed, through which a portion of the food's qi is lost. Therefore, this qi is not available anymore when it comes to digesting the food. Young people, who still have a lot of prenatal qi, usually do not suffer so much from the direct effect of frozen food. Older people, on the other hand, clearly experience—through the feeling of being overly full and bloated—the spleen weakness, which is caused by food that is difficult to digest. Frozen food, especially frozen meat, eventually causes ailments and a weakness of the spleen's qi. This is because, with increasingly difficult

180

Scientific

Findings

regarding

Use of the

Microwave

Oven

digestion, the food now passes slowly through the intestine, which causes the development of putrefactive bacteria, leading to hyperacidity and toxic deposits. From the point of view of TCM, when this happens, a damp heat develops with bloating and foul-smelling stools. In young people, damp heat often manifests as acne. Aside from frozen pizza and similar frozen foods, chocolate, French fries, pork sausage, and cheese are known to cause this troubling skin problem.

Scientific Findings regarding Use of the Microwave Oven

The following quoted statements and research results are drawn from two articles that appeared in the July 1998 issue of the Swiss publication *The Journal of Natural Science*. These articles contain numerous international findings about the damaging effects of microwave radiation on food. Not only can this knowledge help to ban the microwave oven once and for all from the kitchen, but it also can help to spur on government lobbyists concerned with this issue.

The following are typical examples of microwave applications in the food industry:

- *Defrosting* of: Meat, fish, butter, berries. It can be assumed that most perishable foods—like meat, vegetables, and fruits—that are processed into other food products-for example, sausage, ready-made meals, potato chips, and juices-are initially stored frozen and then defrosted with microwave radiation.
- *Cooking:* Bacon, potatoes, pastry, fish, meat, poultry.
- *Drying:* Starchy foods, onions, rice cakes, seaweed.

@ *Vacuum-drying:* Citrus juices, grains, seeds.

The overall problems concerning the microwave can roughly be divided into three categories:

181

Effects of

Processing,

Freezing,

and

Microwaves

@ Effects of the microwave oven on people who are nearby through leaking radiation.

@ Alteration of foods or beverages through microwave radiation.

@ Effects of foods or beverages heated up in the microwave on the organism.

You will find detailed information concerning these three issues in Appendix A of the book. What follows includes only a few selected findings from research conducted on microwave-radiated food and its effect on the organism:

@ In 1989, the Swiss National Fund declined to study the effects of food cooked in the microwave, because, according to them, no need for research in this area existed. So, two researchers financed with their own money a study in which they compared the effects of microwave-radiated food with those of convention- ally prepared food. "Their study . . . proved that food that was prepared in the microwave caused, right after being absorbed, remarkable changes in the blood of the test persons." The authors described these changes as "partially highly significant," and concluded that "the beginning of a pathological process, like, for example, the formation of cancer, existed here."

@ "Proteins, fatty acids, vitamins, and other substances

are, according to scientific research, for the most part not altered chemically. Nevertheless, in the food being cooked, molecular structures are deformed due to the frequent reversion of polarity, and even cellular walls are destroyed. In histological studies, this was observed when carrots and broccoli were cooked in the microwave. In comparison, the cell structures remained intact when they were cooked conventionally. Even the formation of unknown substances caused by microwaves is conceivable. The cells of food that is cooked are polarized destructively through the electrical reversion of polarity caused by the microwaves. Thus, free radicals can come about. All radicals have a special chemical readiness for reaction, and they easily form compounds that are foreign to the cells and destructive to their functioning. Through their reciprocal action with enzymes, they can also affect biological processes."

@ "The fast heating . . . can lead to uneven and barely predictable heat distribution in the foods—with formation of . . . cold and/or hot fields, whereby germs frequently are not inactivated sufficiently. Brief heating of food that is strongly burdened microbially . . . therefore means a clearly higher risk to health . . . As a result, there can be a threat of salmonella poisoning, for example, when chicken meat is not cooked sufficiently."

@ The following experiment was related in a lecture: "Water samples were heated up in the microwave oven and in devices using other sources of energy, and then cooled off again. Kernels of grain were covered with the different water samples, and their sprouting was observed. Of the samples, only the

182

Scientific
Findings
regarding
Use of the
Microwave
Oven

water heated up in the microwave did not cause the grain to germinate."

ⓔ "In the United States, it was proven . . . in 1973 in an animal experiment, that microwaves cause blood cancer."

ⓔ "A study group at Stanford University's School of Medicine in California found that breast milk that is radiated with microwaves at high temperatures (72–98 degrees Celsius) showed a lessening of all resistance factors. It was also found that, at 98 degrees Celsius, the E. coli growth had increased 18 times more than it did in the control group. . . . Already at temperatures of 25–53 degrees Celsius, a significant decrease of the lysozyme content and a greatly increased growth of the E. coli bacteria were observed." From this and other results, the authors concluded that "microwave radiation was not a suitable heating method."

Now let's look at the use of freezing and microwave radiation from the viewpoint of the food chemist Udo Pollmer. In the following, he describes how a problem having to do with the different consistencies of summer and winter cream in butter production is solved.

"In order to guarantee that butter can be spread easily, the milk experts came up with the butter-storage trick. The principle is simple and has to do with taking cream from the opposite respective season. In the winter, the butter is blended with frozen cream that had been stored on a beautiful summer day. And in the summer, winter cream is mixed into the butter. This way, on a regular basis, old fat gets into our fresh German brand-name butter. In order to defrost the milk fat as evenly as possible, microwaves have proven useful. Even though the butter-storage trick requires a lot of energy during the cooling process, the customer saves energy when he spreads the butter." (*Natur*, December 1994)

184

Scientific

Findings

regarding

Use of the

Microwave

Oven

It must be added that the butter is stored and transported frozen, before it ends up as "fresh" butter on the shelves of the supermarkets. This is generally not the case with butter from the organic food stores.

In summary, I want to quote a final statement from an article in *The Journal of Natural Science*, mentioned earlier:

"An individual meal that we heat up in the microwave will not kill us, but after a longer period of time, the altered food will cause so many blockages in the body that it will start to rebel. *One day, the world will wake up and realize that microwaves cause cancer even more than cigarettes do.* When food has been prepared in the microwave oven, it is a creeping death. Superficially, we save some time when we heat up our coffee in the microwave oven in the morning, but whatever time we save takes off time from our own life. Nowhere is there a healing method that can prevent this, as long as we keep using these devices."

Specific Guidelines for Healthy Nutrition

In order to make the selection of food easier for you, the common signs of the most frequent imbalances, together with recommendations to correct them, are summarized below.

Deficiency of Qi/Deficiency of Yang

Deficiency of Qi

The following symptoms point to a deficiency of qi in the spleen:

- Fatigue, especially after a meal, and poor concentration
- Feeling of being overly full, bloating/flatulence, soft stool
- Cold hands and feet
- Cravings for sweets

Deficiency of Yang

These symptoms indicate a deficiency of yang in the kidneys:

- Constantly having cold feet
- Aversion to cold weather and cold beverages
- Frequent urination and/or urinating during the night
- Back pain or stiffness in the early morning, improving with movement

@ Exhaustion, lack of energy, low libido

@ Tremendous need for sleep

The recommendations below are given for a *deficiency of either qi or yang*. When there is a deficiency of yang, the recommendations must be followed more consistently for there to be improvement, because the disorder is more fundamental. The daily warm breakfast is very important, as is at least one other warm meal, along with the use of high-quality warming spices. Refined sugar and all cold foods need to be avoided completely.

For a deficiency of qi or of yang, avoid the following:

@ Foods with a cold thermal effect (especially sour-cold), raw sour-refreshing fruits, and sour-milk products

@ Tropical fruits, uncooked food, refined sugar, and all foods and beverages containing refined sugar

@ Cheese, cream, and milk

@ Frequent meals with bread

@ Frozen food

@ Food prepared or heated up in the microwave

@ Canned food, ready-made meals, margarine

@ Ice-cold beverages

@ Cold drinks with meals

@ Not eating, despite hunger

The following are encouraged:

@ Regularly using fresh ginger, cinnamon, cardamom, and other spices that further digestion

@ Neutral, warm, and hot (in small quantities) foods, especially sweet-neutral vegetables and refreshing cooked vegetables and stewed fruits

- Grains: Especially millet, brown rice, polenta, and oats
- Frequent small quantities (2 tablespoons) of meat, fish, and eggs, preferably in the morning or early afternoon
- Meat, frequently in soups: Beef, chicken, and lamb
- Small quantities of green leafy salad, fresh herbs and sprouts in combination with cooked food; for vegetarians, frequent warming vegetables, legumes, and spices
- A warming breakfast and at least another cooked meal each day
- For breakfast: Grains, cooked for a long time in water or fruit juice, with stewed fruits, cinnamon, nuts; grains with egg, plus vegetables or chicken soup
- Grain coffee, hot water, and tea with spices such as fresh ginger, cinnamon, fennel, and cardamom
- Chewing well, taking time for eating, and enjoying your meals!
- Moving a lot, without overstraining yourself
- Sleeping long enough, but not too long

Dampness with or without Being Overweight

Excess of Yin

An excess of yin means that dampness collects in the tissue due to a qi or yang weakness of the spleen or possibly a yang weakness of the kidneys. The symptoms that follow point to an excess of yin:

- All signs of a deficiency of qi in the spleen
- Water retention in the face, arms, and legs

@ Heavy feeling in the arms and legs

@ Lack of thirst

@ Low spirits

@ Tendency to be overweight

188

Dampness

with or

without

Being

Overweight

Follow the same recommendations as for a deficiency of qi in the spleen, and, in addition, pay attention to the following:

@ Completely forgo milk products (except for butter), uncooked food, honey, and other very sweet foods.

@ Avoid heavy, fatty food, such as fatty sausage and pork.

@ Eat less meals with bread and fast foods.

@ Eat plenty for breakfast and lunch, but avoid big quantities of food and meat for dinner.

@ Roast the grain dry, before cooking, without fat, stirring constantly. Then pour hot water over it and cook it as usual.

@ Regularly use fresh ginger when you cook (especially meat), as well as cardamom and other aromatic spices and herbs.

@ Steam the food in a little water, and add cold-pressed oil and spices at the end.

@ Take cooked-food leftovers from home to work, so that you always have good food available.

@ Do not starve: Eat as soon as you are hungry. You can eat as much cooked vegetables as you wish.

@ Snack on sunflower seeds in-between meals when you are hungry.

These foods and beverages are also advised:

@ Bitter-warm foods, beverages, and spices, such as
   lamb, grain coffee with cardamom
@ Cooked grains
@ Vegetables, briefly steamed in water, with fresh and
   dried herbs and spices
@ Steamed lean meat in small portions, preferably at
   lunch
@ Spice tea, red wine, and hot water

Overweight Due to Dampness and Heat
Damp Heat

Damp heat develops on the basis of a qi weakness of the
spleen, which leads to an excess of yin. The heat factor is
often caused by liver qi stagnation, as stagnation always
leads to heat eventually. Symptoms of damp heat are as
follows:

@ Signs of a deficiency of qi in the spleen and of liver qi
   stagnation, such as having a lump in one's throat,
   tension in the abdomen, and other forms of internal
   tension
@ Water retention
@ Alternately soft stools and constipation
@ Foul-smelling flatulence and stools
@ Dark or cloudy urine
@ Tendency toward one-sided headaches or migraines
@ Acne
@ Aversion to fat, intolerance of food fried in fat
@ Ravenous hunger

Follow the same recommendations as for a deficiency of qi in the spleen, and also adhere to these overall guidelines:

@ Use warming foods and spices moderately.
@ Combine warm, neutral, and refreshing foods in balanced proportions.

In addition, avoid the following:

@ All hot foods, beverages, and spices
@ Fried fat
@ Large quantities of meat, meat dishes in the evening, fried meat, pork and sausage, smoked food
@ Very spicy and heavy food, such as sausage, pizza, and French fries
@ Salty-fatty food, such as chips and salted nuts
@ Sweet-fat food, such as chocolate and cream tarts
@ Milk products, food baked with cheese, and cheese sandwiches
@ Coffee, red wine, and high-proof alcohol
@ Big meals, especially in the evening

These foods and beverages are advised:

@ Simple, light meals, consisting of potatoes, millet, rice, vegetables, and fresh herbs
@ Refreshing vegetables, cut into small pieces, briefly steamed in water
@ Green leafy salads
@ Stewed fruits
@ Small quantities of cooked meat or fish for lunch
@ Hot water, rose-hip tea, green tea, and corn-silk tea

Deficiency of Blood/Deficiency of Yin
Deficiency of Blood

The liver and the heart are affected by a lack of blood. These are the signs of a blood deficiency:

- @ Sensitivity to light, night blindness
- @ Limbs that have fallen asleep
- @ Pale face, pale lips
- @ Emotional vulnerability
- @ Difficulty falling asleep

Deficiency of Yin

A deficiency of yin concerns the kidneys basically. But it can also manifest in the liver, the heart, the stomach, the lungs, and the large intestine. These are the common signs:

- @ Night sweats, hot feet especially at night
- @ Sleep disorders, including waking up in the night
- @ Thirst, a dry mouth
- @ Inner restlessness

The following advice is for a *deficiency of either blood or yin.* Because a yin deficiency is a profound disorder, drying and stimulating foods and beverages such as coffee and Coke must be avoided completely. In addition, refreshing, briefly cooked vegetables should make up the main portion of one's nutrition. Both a lack of yin and a lack of blood always have to do with a deficiency of qi in the spleen.

Follow the same guidelines as for a deficiency of qi in the spleen, and also:

@ Combine warming, neutral, and refreshing foods in balanced portions

In addition, avoid the following:

@ Bitter-warm, bitter-hot, and pungent-hot foods
@ Coffee, black tea, green tea, red wine, and Coke
@ Pungent-warm and pungent-hot food and beverages: Oats, garlic, chili, cayenne, curry, and high-proof alcohol
@ Roasted and barbecued food, extremely browned meat, lamb, or game
@ Intellectual overstrain, reading late into the evening
@ Emotional stress

These foods and beverages are advised:

@ A lot of briefly cooked vegetables; green leafy salads
@ Fresh herbs and sprouts
@ Small amounts of seeds and nuts, especially sunflower seeds and almonds
@ Seaweed
@ Stewed fruits, especially pears with cinnamon and vanilla
@ Grains: Brown rice, wheat semolina, millet, and polenta
@ Potatoes
@ Chicken and freshwater fish in combination with refreshing vegetables
@ Soups
@ Juicy food, steamed in a little water with cold-pressed oil
@ Fruit tea, verbena tea, mint tea, hot water, grape juice with hot water

Excess of Yang

Most frequently an excess of yang occurs in the area of the liver due to emotional stress. The other organs that can be affected by this are the heart and the stomach. These are the signs:

- Strong thirst and hunger
- Sensation of heat
- Reddish face
- Dark urine, dark and hard stool
- Irritability
- Easily losing one's temper
- Restlessness, strong need for activity
- Sleep disorders

With an excess of yang, avoid the following:

- Foods with a hot thermal effect; also, for the most part, warming foods and beverages
- Strongly browned and barbecued food
- Meat, sausage, and eggs, in large quantities
- Pork
- Oat flakes
- Very spicy food and pungent spices, like chili, curry, and garlic
- High-proof alcohol, red wine, coffee, and Coke
- Stress and lack of sleep

The following are encouraged:

- Light meals with a lot of briefly cooked, refreshing vegetables, mushrooms, green leafy salads, fresh herbs and sprouts

@ Neutral and refreshing foods, small quantities of cold foods

@ On a regular basis, sour-refreshing food, like stewed fruit and very ripe fruit

@ Rice, millet, wheat, polenta, potatoes

@ Steamed fresh fish, seaweed

@ Fruit tea, verbena tea (vervain), hot water, fruit juices with hot water

Applying Different Kinds
of Taste

A healthy, balanced diet based on the seasons and our own needs not only is good for us but also keeps us from becoming bored and too set in our ways. Just as we change as we go through the different phases of our life, the needs of the body change over the course of the seasons. Use your five senses, and perceive what is happening around you; then it will be much easier for you to pick up on the signals of your body, which constantly tries to adapt to new situations.

For example, if you find yourself craving sweets, don't go for the first sweet food that comes to mind. Take a look at the food lists in Appendix B, and eat for one to two weeks as many sweet, rich-in-qi foods as possible. Good choices are pumpkin, carrots, millet, dried fruits, and nuts. Strengthen the spleen with beef broth, and allow yourself a warm breakfast. You will be surprised how fast the craving for chocolate and other sweets will disappear when your body gets what it truly needs.

A young woman who was a writer came to me for nutritional counseling. She was so exhausted all the time that she had to take an afternoon nap every day. As a vegetarian, she thought she had to eat a lot of milk products in order to supply her body with sufficient protein. Thus, she ate a pound of cottage cheese every day. She couldn't believe it when I told her to forgo milk products altogether for a while. I also recommended some earth foods and vegetable-protein suppliers, and she was willing to try them.

She called me after three weeks and reported that she hadn't had any milk products at all and had felt much better. Then she called again a few days later, informing me that she had eaten a couple of slices of bread with some cream cheese just to see if that made any difference. "After that," she said, "I felt completely blocked. My body became so heavy that I had to lie down immediately and had to sleep."

This strong reaction, the result of a spleen qi weakness, is not the rule. But it does show how easy it can be to find out for ourselves what is good for us when we question our daily eating habits and make a change. Try going back to your old habits every now and then, so that you can see how much better you feel when you eat the foods that are right for you. When you have not eaten any refined white sugar for several weeks, a slice of cream tart might seem way too sweet after the third bite.

196

Cooking
with the
Five
Different
Tastes

Cooking with the Five Different Tastes

In order to be able to eat a balanced diet all year long, there are some simple guidelines concerning taste that make the selection of food easier:

@ The five different tastes should nourish the organs in a balanced manner. The more flavors there are in a meal, the better the organs are cared for. If you prepare meals with several spices and herbs, you have achieved this goal. Or you can simply combine different kinds of vegetables such as carrots, kohlrabi, and red beets, along with millet or polenta. In a balanced meal, every taste is clearly noticeable, but none predominates.

- Pay attention to the colors. A variety of colors and a pleasing aroma stimulate the digestive juices and prepare the stomach for the food. A meal that contains all five colors stimulates qi and looks very appetizing. Try yellow peppers, celery, and zucchini or broccoli. Another good combination is carrots or red peppers and black seaweed. Or sprinkle the dish with black sesame seeds.

- Earth foods are an exception. They can be combined without other flavors, and the organs are still nourished in a balanced manner, as the mild-sweet taste is harmonious on its own and distributes the qi throughout the entire body. Serve a beef goulash with polenta and green string beans, or simply millet along with carrots with roasted hazelnuts.
- Aromatic herbs and spices play an important role. Caraway seeds, nutmeg, thyme, sage, marjoram, and fresh ginger not only give the dish flavor, but they also make even heavy dishes containing legumes, meat, or fat more digestible. Fresh herbs, briefly cooked, that are sprinkled over the dish before the meal is served have the same effect. Fresh basil, oregano, chives, chervil, and watercress are good replacements in dishes for the usual garlic or cream sauce.

Cooking according to the Season

In order to use or balance the influences of the seasons, the respective tastes and thermal effects can be emphasized. However, it would be an oversimplification to say that we should predominantly eat sour foods in the spring, bitter foods in the summer, sweet foods in the late summer, pungent foods in the fall, and salty foods in the winter. It's a little more complicated than that, as you'll see.

- ◉ Qi and wind predominate in the *spring*, and there is a danger of dryness. Spring is the time to strengthen the liver and the gallbladder. The foods preferred now have a portion of wood, in order to complete, restore, or preserve the bodily fluids. Examples are green vegetables, leafy vegetables, sprouts, fresh herbs, and ripe fruit. In addition, wheat, spelt, small quantities of sour-milk products, and poultry are used more frequently than usual. After the rich winter diet of meat and legumes, light vegetable and grain dishes are now called for, as they detoxify the body and help to give it more mobility.

- ◉ In the *summer*, heat is the dominating temperature. This is the time to use more yin-enhancing cooking methods, as well as refreshing vegetables, mushrooms, steamed tomatoes, leafy salads, sprouts, fruits, and tofu, and less meat. Make salads with cooked vegetables, as they are easier to digest than uncooked food. Hot beverages and food make summer heat tolerable, because the discrepancy between the temperature inside and that outside is kept minimal. This is one of the reasons why, in hot countries, pungent spices are used also in the summer. In addition, the organism is especially sensitive in the hot season to ice-cold food and beverages, as they shock the stomach and the spleen. Therefore, consuming ice-cold food and drinks should be avoided also in the summer. At first, a hot cup of fruit tea or lemon water or a pungent dish can bring on a wave of heat, but, after that, the heat outside becomes much more tolerable.

@ In the *fall*, it's generally dry. Inside the body, the fluids withdraw, so the lungs and the large intestine tend to be dry, manifesting as a dry cough or constipation. Rice, radishes, and white vegetables such as kohlrabi and cauliflower strengthen and protect the metal organs. At the same time, the organism needs to be prepared for the cold season by strengthening the body's resistance. Leeks, onions, fresh ginger, other pungent spices, and lamb are all good for this. The protein portion of the meal can now be increased again with meat, fish, eggs, legumes, and nuts. Hearty soups and stews provide a nourishing basis for withstanding unfavorable weather conditions.

@ In the *winter*, cold dominates. Yang-enhancing cooking methods and warming foods, spices, and herbs are now preferred. But very warm food always needs to be balanced with refreshing vegetables and winter salads. The winter is the time to build up reserves, especially when it comes to the bones, which profit in the cold season from an abundant supply of minerals. Seaweed, for example, has a high mineral content and goes very well in soups, stews, and dishes with legumes. Nuts are also rich in minerals and can be used to enhance salads, stewed fruits, and vegetable dishes. Walnuts are said to be a kidney tonic; eaten regularly in small quantities, they strengthen the yang of the kidneys.

In order to cook according to the seasons, however, you must make a few adjustments in your calendar. Where the "beginning of spring" is marked on the calendar, it has already been spring, in reality, for thirty-six days.

To determine the beginning and the end of the seasons this new way, proceed as follows: Calculate thirty-six days back and thirty-six days ahead from the usual beginning of spring, summer, fall, and winter. Then you will have a more accurate beginning and end of the respective season, which lasts seventy-two days. Mark these key dates on your calendar, and pay attention to what is happening on the first days of the new season outside with the air and nature. For example, you will probably see that around mid-February as the birds are starting to chirp again and the first shoots are coming out of the snow, it will be about thirty-six days before the official beginning of spring on the twenty-first of March. Since I have used this time calculation, I am happy every year that spring begins so early for me, and I enjoy looking for all its signs.

You will notice that there are about eighteen days left in-between each season of seventy-two days. This is what's called the "dojo time." The earth element predominates during these eighteen days, forming a transition from each season to the next. This time is especially suitable for strengthening the spleen and the stomach with help from the earth foods and for nourishing the organism with sweet and yellow food rich in carbohydrates.

The Little Dot on the "i"

I also want to share with you a special feature of the Five-Elements Plan that evokes stunning taste experiences while also making the food more digestible.

Cooking according to the Cycle of the Elements

Cooking a stew, a meat soup, or a dish consisting of several vegetables is the best way for you to become familiar with this cooking method. The essence of this technique is *adding the individual ingredients in the sequence of the generative cycle.* For this, it is of course necessary to know to which elements the foods and the spices belong.

I resisted this method myself for a long time, as it seemed obscure and excessive to me, even though I was told again and again that dishes prepared in this manner have a highly energetic effect and always taste delicious. When I began to teach Chinese dietetics myself, I finally took the step in finding out what this method was all about.

The place where I first tried it was well chosen. At that time, I often spent weekends at a former farm in the Allgäu that some friends were rebuilding into a beautiful seminary house. A lot of people came to help on the weekend, and everyone was grateful when they had something warm to eat for lunch. Thus, I looked into the storage room and developed a stew according to the five elements. But before I began cooking, I wrote down the allocation of the ingredients in the right sequence on a piece of paper. Then the cooking could begin. Picture this:

The pot is heated up first; I am now in the fire element. Next oil is added, earth element; then carrots, also earth. *In one element, different ingredients of that same element can be added.* Now I wait a moment and stir, before adding the leek and kohlrabi, cut into small pieces, into the metal element. The vegetables are now browned. In the water element that follows, I add a pinch of salt, stirring again. As the recipe does not call for any foods from the wood element, and *I must not skip an element,* I simply add some lemon juice. A generous pinch of thyme and a glass of red wine represent the fire element; after adding them, I stir once more. Now I wait until the vegetables are almost fully cooked. At this point, it's time for the earth element again with a spoonful of honey or a little bit of heavy cream, then the metal element with pepper and nutmeg, and finally the water element as I season the stew with a little more salt.

The art lies in using the spices in the correct quantities. If you forget a spice, you must continue the cycle until you reach the element of the missing spice, by adding *very small quantities* of the respective subsequent elements. It is also possible to go back a step if you inadvertently skip an element, *but you can go back only one step.* If, for example, you realize in the water element, just after adding salt, that you forgot pepper, you can go back and add the pepper. However, so that you do not skip the water element, you need to add another tiny pinch of salt before proceeding to the wood element.

It is said that the organs of the element where you end up in the cooking process receive the most qi. Should you want to strengthen the kidneys, for example, the last ingredient should be from the water element. This can be a tiny pinch of salt. Should you want to strengthen the spleen, it is best to end with the earth element. However, I don't take this rule too seriously myself, as any dish cooked according to the cycle of the elements will have a special energetic quality, and I like to leave which element to use last up to my intuition.

Going through the cycle several times may be a good way to get the best flavoring. But it depends on the dish you are preparing. With some dishes, just one or two cycles are best. I discovered this the first time I tried the stew, thinking I would need to go through the cycle several times to give the meal a tolerable taste. But even though I went through the cycle only twice, and used very simple ingredients, the meal was a tremendous success, and no one had to add anymore seasoning. As a side dish, I served brown rice with roasted sunflower seeds. After bringing the pots into the dining room, I went outside for a few minutes to get some fresh air and cool off from the heat of the stove. When I returned, I received an enthusiastic applause.

Since then, I have had many similar experiences. And each time I am surprised how tasty a very simple meal can be and what a good mood develops around the table, when the dish was prepared in the sequence of the elements. From students in my courses and clients whom I've counseled, I've received again and again the same confirmation—that meals that are cooked following the generative cycle taste absolutely delicious and are very digestible. I even prepare my salad dressings, which are especially important to me, in this sequence.

Several participants in my training groups who were willing to experiment cooked the same meal twice: once following the generative cycle, and the second time in the sequence to which they were accustomed. Then they asked their family or their guests which version was the better one. The assessment was always unmistakable: The meal cooked in the sequence of the generative cycle tasted the best.

One of these participants showed me a handwritten little book with the recipes of her grandmother. Astonishingly, the sequence of the ingredients in most of the recipes corresponded to that of the generative cycle. For me, this was another validation of the universal principles underlying Chinese dietetics.

If you want to try cooking this way yourself, some additional information is necessary:

- *A hot pot is a fire element.* When you now add fat, you are in the earth element.
- *Raw onions are in the metal element.* But if they are fried, they lose their pungent taste and become sweet, so you are *back to the earth element.* Now you must use a pungent ingredient again, in order not to skip the metal element.
- *Cold water is obviously a water element.* Therefore, when you put a pot with cold water onto the stove, the first ingredient that you need to use must be either a water or a wood element. But if you wait until the *water becomes hot,* or you *add hot water to a dish,* then you are in the *fire element,* and the next ingredient must be fire or earth.

In order to make it easier for you to cook this way, always write down at the beginning the sequence of the ingredients. The foods listed according to their element in

Appendix B will be a helpful reference for this. If you are not sure where a spice belongs, taste a little bit and go by the predominant flavor. It can also be helpful to stick small colored dots, according to the colors of the elements, onto your spice jars.

So, enjoy your shopping and your experiments, and always bon appétit!

Appendix A:

Further Results of Microwave Research

I have gathered a great deal of information regarding the danger of microwave ovens over the past several years. For the most part, this data comes from the same sources that *The Journal of Natural Science,* which I quoted earlier, also used as a basis for its articles. Yet I have not published it until now, because I knew that several scientists who had dared to do that ended up revoking their statements, as they were afraid of losing their jobs and were concerned about their well-being and the safety of their families. In Europe, for example, the following occurred.

As alluded to previously, in 1989 in Switzerland the environmental biologist Dr. Hans Hertel researched the effects of food radiated with microwaves on the human organism. The publication of his results in various media caused many consumers to feel quite insecure. Certainly the makers of microwave ovens felt insecure. Because of a complaint filed by a trade association representing electrical devices, the Swiss Federal Constitutional Court issued a prohibition against Dr. Hertel in 1994. Among other things, he was prohibited from making "the assertion that food prepared in the microwave oven was damaging to health and led to changes in the blood of its consumers, indicating a pathological disorder and possibly the beginning of a carcinogenic (cancer-producing) process." But on August 25, 1998, the European Tribunal for Human Rights decided that Dr. Hertel was allowed to enter his scientific findings on the danger of microwave ovens into the public debate. As a result of this verdict, the Swiss Federal Constitutional Court had to lift his prohibition. This development should give us hope that the shocking results of his research now finally can be made accessible to the general public.

So that you can better picture the situation yourself, I quote in the following a number of important points from two articles in the July 1998 issue of *The Journal of Natural Science*.

Physical Principle of Microwave Radiation

A fundamental effect of microwave treatment is the quick heating of food achieved through friction heat. "The essential part of the oven is the so-called magnetron, which produces an alternating-current field. The high-frequency reversion of polarity in this electromagnetic field forces the molecules in the foods—especially the water dipoles, but also the amino acids, lipides, and proteins—to orient themselves constantly in this field according to their charge. In other words, they swing back and forth up to 2.5 billion times per second, thus producing the friction heat. The food is heated this way from the inside, while the cooking dishes and the oven casing, which do not absorb any microwaves, remain cold."

Safety Limits and Leaking Radiation

"Since the first usage of microwaves during the Second World War, people in the West have known of their harmfulness in regards to biological systems. Russian researchers had already in the thirties investigated the effects of microwave radiation of little performance density on the central nervous system. But the safety regulations that resulted from this and that were extremely strict were not taken seriously by the Western colleagues in the field, and still in the sixties were exceeded a thousandfold."

"The U.S. Committee for Radiation Protection, NCRP, made it known at the end of the eighties that an increased number of birth defects occurs in children of women who work with microwave ovens."

"A study of microwave household devices in Washington, D.C., and two states of the United States showed that, at the end of the eighties, cooking, defrosting, and barbecuing devices were emitting a radiation intensity 25 percent higher than the safety limit of 10mW/cm2, even when their doors were closed. During a merchandise test, 24 out of 30 microwave ovens had to be singled out as being too dangerous. The radiation leaks of these devices reached up to 20mW/cm2."

"A housewife can suffer easily from eye damage by standing every day in front of an invisible radiation leak of her cooking device when the oven is installed at the height of her face; she could possibly even become blind."

"The *Berliner Stiftung Warentest* [equivalent to Consumer Report], for example, found in 1990, when they tested microwave ovens for their technical safety, that none of the microwave ovens was leak-proof."

"The Swiss Federal Office of Health, on the other hand, expressed its view in 1992 concerning the subject of 'radiation leaks' as follows: 'The microwave radiation that escapes from technically perfectly functioning and expertly used microwave household cooking devices does not pose any health danger for human beings, not even for people who particularly need to be protected, like, for example, pregnant women and small children. Fire and gas, however, pose much more important danger factors.' "

Thermal and Non-thermal Effects

"Aside from *thermal*, i.e., heat-causing, effects, one must also reckon with *non-thermal* effects of microwave radiation, that is, reciprocal actions between microwave radiation and structures in living organisms that are not contingent upon friction heat. Whereas in Russia non-thermal effects are taken into consideration as well for setting the limiting values, in other countries, like Germany, for example, thermal effects are considered exclusively. In comparison to other countries, Germany is the leader when it comes to how freely microwaves are allowed to put a strain on the population."

"In a report issued by the Institute for Radiation Hygiene of the German Federal Public Health Department (BGA) from 1980, in which 16 reports were compared and evaluated, the following effects of microwave radiation, thermal and non-thermal, were described:

- Activity changes of enzymes and influence on enzymatic processes,
- Influence on the thyroid glands and suprarenal gland and its hormones,
- Effects on the combination and/or function of blood components,
- Influence on cell growth and chromosome changes,
- Turbidity of the eye lenses (cataracts),
- Influence on the concentration and/or functioning of blood components and hormones in the brain."

Research from Germany and Russia

A forensic research document, containing results from numerous studies, is in the archives of the Atlantis Educational Center in Portland, Oregon. The author William Kopp had worked there from 1977 until 1979, and had collected comprehensive material about the harmfulness of microwaves. Because of this, he came under so much pressure that he changed his name and disappeared. As regards the contents of the document:

From 1942 to 1943, the German Wehrmacht conducted studies at Humboldt University in Berlin regarding the usage of microwave ovens for cooking during the Barbarossa campaign in Russia. Based on the results, which proved the harmfulness to health through consuming food heated up by microwaves, the devices were not used.

"After World War Two had ended, the allies confiscated the medical research papers, documents, and devices. . . . The Soviet Union continued to do research independently." The consequence was that in 1976 the Soviet Union legally banned the usage of microwave ovens. "They also published an international warning concerning the possible biological effects and harmfulness to the environment that the usage of these or similar electronic devices could cause."

Since 1957, the Russians have been conducting research at the Institutes for Radio-Technology in Kinsk and Rajasthan. "In most cases, the foods that were used for the analysis were exposed to microwaves with an efficiency current density of 100 kilowatt/cm3/second, the quantity that, at that time, was still considered acceptable for a normal, healthy consumption of food."

A list of consequences, covering twenty-eight points,

that were determined by the German and Russian researchers can be subdivided into three categories:

1. Cancer-causing effects
2. Destruction of the food's nutritional value
3. Biological effects of exposure to microwaves

Selected points from each category follow.

1. Cancer-causing effects

- Formation of d-nitrosodiethanolamin (a carcinogen) was found in pre-prepared meat heated up sufficiently to guarantee hygienic food consumption.
- Destabilizing of active biomolecular protein combinations occurred.
- Formation of carcinogens occurred in the protein-hydrolysat combinations of milk and grains.
- Alteration of elementary nutrients that caused functional disorders in the digestive tract was linked to the decomposition of microwave-radiated food.
- As a result of the chemical alterations in the foods, functional disorders in the lymphatic system were noticed. Through this, the body's resistance to certain forms of neoplasma (new cancer-like formations in tissue) is reduced.
- The consumption of microwave-radiated nutrition led to an increased number of cancer cells in the blood serum.
- Cancer-causing *free radicals* developed in certain molecular forms of trace elements in vegetables, especially in raw root vegetables.
- In a large number of people, food radiated by microwaves caused statistically significant cancer-like

lumps in the stomach and in the digestive tract, in addition to a general degeneration of the periphery cell tissue, with a gradual collapse of the functions of the digestion and excretion system.

2. *Destruction of the food's nutritional value:* Microwave radiation was found to cause a significant reduction in the nutritional value of all examined foods. The following are the most significant findings:

- Reduction in the bio-availability (capability of the body to absorb a nutrient and make it available at the place of action) of the B-complex, C, and E vitamins, the essential minerals, and fatty substances in all food products.
- Loss of 60 to 90 percent of the vital energy of all tested foods.
- Decrease in the nutritional value of nucleo-proteins in meat.

3. *Biological effects of exposure to microwaves*

- Reduction of the life-energy field in people exposed to switched-on microwave ovens, with long-lasting ramifications.
- Degeneration of the cellular potential while the device is being used, especially in the blood and lymph fluids.
- Degeneration and destabilization of the ability to utilize nutrients, which is activated by light energy.
- Degeneration of nerve circulation and the electrical stimulation transmission in the cerebrum.
- Destabilization and disturbance of hormone production and maintenance in both men and women.
- Disturbance of brain-wave patterns (alpha, theta, and delta waves) in people exposed to microwave fields.

@ Through disturbance of the brain waves, negative effects such as loss of memory, poor concentration, lower level of emotional tolerance, slowdown of the thinking processes, and sleep disorders were noticed. These effects were observed in a significantly higher percentage in people who were exposed continuously to radiation of electromagnetic fields from microwave ovens as well as microwave transmitters.

The Swiss Study

In a special 1992 edition of the Swiss magazine *Raum & Zeit*, in an article titled "Hands Off the Microwave Oven!" the Ehlers Publishing Company published the results of the earlier-mentioned study by the Swiss biologist Dr. Hans Hertel. For the study, the test persons were given raw milk, conventionally cooked milk, pasteurized milk, milk cooked in the microwave oven, as well as raw vegetables, conventionally cooked vegetables, vegetables cooked in the microwave oven, and frozen vegetables defrosted in the microwave. What follow are excerpts from the article.

"Directly before and in defined intervals after the food consumption, the test persons' blood was taken and checked for certain criteria.

"The result: The food (milk and vegetables) that was heated, defrosted, or cooked in the microwave oven caused in the blood of the test persons significant changes. Among them were a decrease of all hemoglobin values and an increase of the hematocrites, the leucozytes, and the cholesterine values, especially of the HDL and of the LDL portions. A momentarily stronger decrease of the lymphozytes was noticeable in all vegetables prepared in

the microwave oven, when compared with all other variations.

"With the illuminating power of luminescent bacteria,
a significant connection between the absorption of technical microwave energy and of radiated food products and
the illuminating power that could be measured afterward
in the blood serum of the test persons was determined.

"The measured effects of the microwaves by way of
food on human beings showed, in contrast to nonradiated
food, changes in the blood, which hint at the beginning of
a pathogenic process, just as is the case at the onset of
cancer."

Appendix B:

Foods Listed according to the Five Elements

Element	Hot	Warm	Neutral	Refreshing	Cold
WOOD					
Sour, leads to the inside, preserves fluids		*Fruit:* Kumquats Pomegranates *Meat:* Chicken *Herbs/Spices:* Parsley Vinegar *Beverages:* Cherry juice	*Grains:* Bulgar Couscous Spelt *Fruit* Blackberries Raspberries *Beverages:* Rose-hip tea	*Grains:* Wheat *Vegetables:* Alfalfa sprouts Legume sprouts Sauerkraut *Fruit:* Apples, sour Blueberries Bilberries Cherries, sour Gooseberries Mandarin oranges Red currants Strawberries *Meat:* Duck *Milk Products:* Cottage cheese Cream cheese Kefir Sour cream *Beverages:* Balm-mint tea Champagne Hibiscus tea Mallow tea Sparkling wine Wheat beer White wine	*Grains:* Wheat bran Wheat sprouts *Vegetables:* Mung-bean sprouts Sorrel Tomatoes *Fruit:* Kiwi Lemons Pineapple Rhubarb *Milk Products:* Yogurt

Element	Hot	Warm	Neutral	Refreshing	Cold
FIRE					
Bitter, leads	*Meat:*	*Vegetables:*	*Grains:*	*Grains:*	
downward,	All grilled	Brussels	Amaranth	Buckwheat	
stimulates	meats	sprouts	Quinoa	*Vegetables/*	
digestion	Goat	*Milk*	Rye	*Salads:*	
	Lamb	*Products:*	*Vegetables/*	Artichoke	
	Mutton	Goat's milk	*Salads:*	Chicory	
	Beverages:	Goat's milk	Endive	Dandelion	
	Bitter liqueur	cheese	lettuce	Parsnips	
	Cognac	*Herbs/*	Iceberg	Radicchio	
	Hot spicy	*Spices:*	lettuce	Rucola	
	wine	Basil (f)	Red beets	Salad	
		Cacao	Stinging	greens	
		Fenugreek	nettle	*Fruit:*	
		Juniper	*Beverages:*	Elderberries	
		berries	Black tea	Grapefruit	
		Oregano (f)		Quince	
		Paprika		*Herbs:*	
		Poppy		Sage (f)	
		Rosemary (f)		*Beverages:*	
		Savory (f)		Dark beer	
		Thyme (f)		Green tea	
		Turmeric		Water, hot	
		Beverages:			
		Coffee			
		Grain coffee			
		Red wine			

Element	Hot	Warm	Neutral	Refreshing	Cold
EARTH					
Sweet,		*Grains:*	*Grains:*	*Grains:*	*Vegetables:*
distributes qi		Rice, sweet	Millet	Barley	Cucumber
in all directions,		*Vegetables:*	Polenta	*Vegetables:*	*Fruit:*
nourishes and		Chestnuts	*Vegetables:*	Asparagus	Honeydew
moistens		Fennel	Cabbage,	Broccoli	melon
		Onion, fried	red/white	Cabbage,	Mango
		Sweet	Carrots	Chinese	Papaya
		potatoes	Green	Cauliflower	Watermelon
		Fruit:	beans	Celery, bulb	
		Apricots	Kohlrabi	and stick	
		Cherries,	Peas (f)	Champignon	
		sweet	Potatoes	Chard	
		Currants	Savoy	Comfrey	
		Peaches	Turnips	Eggplant	
		Raisins	Yams	Pepper	
		Sultana	Fruit:	Spinach	
		Salad Oils:	Dates (d)	Zucchini	
		Pumpkinseed	Figs (f, d)	*Fruit:*	
		oil	Plums (d)	Apples,	
		Rape oil	*Meat:*	sweet	
		Soy oil	Beef	Bananas	
		Spices:	Milk	Grapes,	
		Cinnamon	*Products:*	red/green	
		Nuts/	Butter	Pears	
		Seeds:	Cheese	*Soy*	
		Coconut	Milk	*Products:*	
		Peanuts	*Spices:*	Soy milk	
		Pine nuts	Saffron	Tofu	
		Walnuts	Vanilla	*Milk*	
		Other:	*Sweeteners:*	*Products:*	
		Coconut	Cane sugar	Heavy	
		milk	Honey	cream,	
		Beverages:	Malt	sweet	
		Fennel tea	Molasses	*Salad Oils:*	
		Honey wine	*Nuts/Seeds:*	Linseed oil	
		Liqueur	Almonds	Olive oil	
		Port wine	Hazelnuts	Sesame oil	
			Pistachio	Sunflower	
			nuts	oil	
			Pumpkin	Wheat-germ	
			seeds	oil	

Element	Hot	Warm	Neutral	Refreshing	Cold
EARTH (continued)					
			Sesame seeds	*Herbs/Spices:*	
			Sunflower seeds	Tarragon (f)	
			Other:	*Sweeteners:*	
			Eggs	Refined white sugar	
			Mushroom, forest	Syrup (all kinds)	
			Mushroom, Shiitake	*Nuts:*	
			Beverages:	Cashew nuts	
			Grape juice, red/white	*Other:*	
			Liquorice tea	Avocado Champignon	
				Beverages:	
				Apple juice	
				Pear juice	

Element	Hot	Warm	Neutral	Refreshing	Cold
METAL					
Pungent, leads upward and outward, moves and dissolves stagnation	*Meat:* Venison *Milk Products:* Moldy cheese *Spices:* Cayenne pepper Chili Curry Garlic Ginger (d) Pepper Pimento	*Grains:* Oats *Vegetables:* Horseradish Leeks Onions, raw Spring onions *Meat:* Partridge Pheasant Roe Wild boar Wild hare	*Grains:* Rice *Vegetables:* Radishes, black *Meat:* Goose Quail Rabbit, wild Turkey, hen	*Vegetables:* Radishes, red/white Radish sprouts Watercress *Meat:* Rabbit, domesticated *Beverages:* Peppermint tea	

Element	Hot	Warm	Neutral	Refreshing	Cold

METAL (continued)

	Beverages:	*Milk*			
	Alcohol,	*Products:*			
	high-proof	Munster			
	Yogi tea	cheese			
		Beverages:			
		Rice wine			
		(sake)			
		Herbs/			
		Spices:			
		Basil (d)			
		Caraway			
		Cardamom			
		Chives (f, d)			
		Cloves			
		Coriander			
		Cumin			
		Dill (f, d)			
		Ginger (f)			
		Laurel (bay)			
		Lovage (f, d)			
		Marjoram (f, d)			
		Masala			
		Mugwort (d)			
		Mustard			
		seeds			
		Nutmeg			
		Oregano (d)			
		Rosemary (d)			
		Savory (d)			
		Star anise			
		Tarragon (d)			
		Thyme (d)			

Element	Hot	Warm	Neutral	Refreshing	Cold
WATER Salty, leads down deep, strengthens bones, dissolves stagnation		*Fish:* Anchovy Cod Eel Lobster Plaice Shrimp Smoked Fish Tuna *Meat/ Cold Cuts:* Ham Pickled, smoked, salted, and dried meat Salami	*Legumes:* Aduki beans Broad beans Lentils Peas (d) Soy beans, yellow/ black *Fish:* Carp Perch Salmon Trout *Meat:* Pork *Other:* Miso	*Legumes:* Chickpeas Mung beans *Seafood:* Oysters Squid *Other:* Olives Umeboshi plums *Beverages:* Mineral water Water, cold	*Seaweed:* Hijiki Kombu Nori Wakame *Seafood:* Caviar Crab (round shell with claws) Crawfish Mussels *Spices:* Salt Soy sauce (Tamari, Shoyu) *Other:* Agar-agar

Note: f = fresh, d = dried

Bibliography

Chinese Dietary Therapy

Da Liu. *The Tao of Health and Longevity.* New York: Schocken Books, 1979

Flaws, Bob and Wolfe, Honora. *Prince Wen Hui's Cook: Chinese Dietary Therapy.* Brookline, MA: Paradigm Pub., 1983

Lu, Henry C. *Chinese System of Food Cures: Prevention & Remedies.* New York: Sterling Pub., 1986

Lu, Henry C. *Chinese System of Foods for Health and Healing.* New York: Sterling Pub., 2000

Lu, Henry C. *Legendary Chinese Healing Herbs.* New York: Sterling Pub., 1991

Pitchford, Paul. *Healing with Whole Foods: Oriental Traditions and Modern Nutrition.* Berkley: North Atlantic Books, 1993

Traditional Chinese Medicine

Connelly, Dianne M. *Traditional Acupuncture: The Law of the Five Elements.* Columbia, MD: Centre for Traditional Acupuncture Inc., 1989

Kaptchuk, Ted. *The Web That Has No Weaver.* New York: Congdon & Weed, 1983

Eastern Psychology

Hammer, Leon M.D. *Dragon Rises Red Bird Flies: Psychology and Chinese Medicine.* New York: Station Hill Press, Inc., 1990

Watts, Alan. *Psychotherapy East & West.* New York: Vintage Books, a Division of Random House, 1975

Politics and Ethics of Food

Anthelme, Jean. *Brillat-Savarin: The Physiology of Taste or Meditations of Transcendental Gastronomy.* San Francisco, CA: North Point Press, 1986

Hightower, Jim. *Eat Your Heart Out: How Food Profiteers Victimize the Consumer.* New York: Vintage Books, a Division of Random House, 1976

Shopping Guides for Whole Food

East West Journal Editors. *Shopper's Guide to Natural Foods.* Garden City Park, NY: Avery Pub. Group, 1987

Wittenberg, Magaret M. *Experiencing Quality: A Shopper's Guide to Whole Foods.* Austin, TX: Whole Foods Market, 1987

Index

About the Author

In her study of traditional Chinese medicine, Barbara Temelie, a native of Germany, has devoted herself specifically to the subjects of nutrition, healthy lifestyle, and Eastern psychology. The ideas she expresses in this book, initially published in the German-speaking countries of Europe, are not only based on her understanding of TCM but also on her many years of working as a nutritional counselor. Her practice includes individual diagnosis based on the principles of TCM and detailed instruction in the practical application of the Five-Elements Plan. In addition to working with individual clients, she conducts intensive training courses in the Five-Elements Plan and teaches cooking classes for the daily application of Chinese dietetics. Along with her colleagues, she also conducts a one-year training program in nutritional counseling. Other books by Barbara Temelie are *The Five-Element Cookbook* and *The Five-Element Diet for Mother and Child*, both written with Beatrice Trebuth and published in Germany.